Eunice Dyke

Health Care Pioneer

From Pioneer Public Health Nurse
to Advocate for the Aged

by Marion Royce

Dundurn Press
Toronto and Charlottetown
1983

Editor: Bernice Lever
Design and production: Ron and Ron Design Photography
Typesetting: Computype
Printing: Editions Marquis, Montmagny, Quebec

The publication of this book was made possible by support from several sources. The author and publisher wish to acknowledge the generous assistance and ongoing support of the Canada Council and the Ontario Arts Council.

J. Kirk Howard, Publisher

Canadian Cataloguing in Publication Data

Royce, Marion V. (Marion Victoria), 1901-
  Eunice Dyke, health care pioneer

(Dundurn lives; 3)
Bibliography: p.
Includes index.
ISBN 0-919670-67-9 (bound). — ISBN 0-919670-64-4 (pbk.)

1. Dyke, Eunice, 1883-1969. 2. Public health nurses
— Canada — Biography. 3. Aged — Services for —
Canada — Biography. I. Title. II. Series.

RT37.D9R6   610.73'4'0924   C83-098544-1

Eunice Dyke

Health Care Pioneer

From Pioneer Public Health Nurse
to Advocate for the Aged

In Memory of My Two Sisters

Jean 1904-1982

and

Catherine 1909-1972

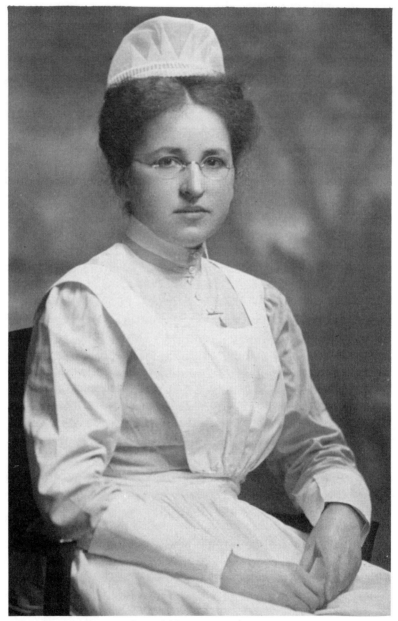

Eunice Henrietta Dyke, 1909

Contents

Preface

It was photographs of early public health nurses in Toronto that led me to Eunice Henrietta Dyke. She, I later learned, was one of those young women in tailored suits, with fitted jackets and floor-length skirts, wearing sensible hats and white blouses, complete with four-in-hand ties, and carrying black 'doctor' bags. The nurse might be standing at the door of a poor dwelling talking with a woman plainly in awe of so austere, yet kindly a person; or, dressed in a white cover-all, weighing babies in a clinic while anxious mothers looked on; or again, teaching a group of small girls how to bathe a baby, obviously a rather large doll. Some shots were taken in a classroom where the nurse was talking on a health subject, or assisting a doctor as he examined children hoping to go to camp. The photographs piqued my curiosity. Here was a dimension of the nursing profession that expanded my image of the traditional nurse. On enquiry, I was told that the Nursing Division of the Department of Public Health had kept scrupulous records of its work of which 'Miss Dyke' had laid the foundation.

So began a search of many facets in which I have depended strongly on those and other records in the City of Toronto Archives, whose staff have been helpful far beyond the claims of duty. I have had access, also, to other archival collections in the city: the University of Toronto Archives, the Library of the Academy of Medicine, hospital and church archives, files of the Canadian Red Cross Society and papers of the Family Service Bureau of Metropolitan Toronto. In addition, the Reference Library of Metropolitan Toronto and the Municipal Library have turned up useful sources, including newspapers on microfilm and contemporary pamphlets. In Ottawa, I consulted records of the Library of the Canadian Nurses Association, and papers of the Canadian Welfare Council in the Public Archives of Canada. Requests for information sent to Simmons College, Boston, and to the

Archives of the Rockefeller Foundation in Poughkeepsie, New York, were graciously answered, and an enquiry about conditions in Saskatchewan during the early years of the Depression brought a generous response from the Saskatchewan Archives Board in the University of Regina.

Later in her life, Miss Dyke, aware of the rapid demographic changes in Canadian society, devoted her energies to emerging needs of the elderly. They were living longer and had begun to represent a growing proportion of the population. Yet little consideration had been given to their health and welfare and how they were to maintain dignity and self-respect. Not even the helping professions, medicine and social work, had come to grips with the changing circumstances of their lives. Working with a group of older women, later including men also, she became increasingly aware of these shortcomings in social organization. A doer as well as a thinker, she was instrumental in founding the first association of senior citizens in Toronto, and she spent her last active years giving birth to ideas that forecast later developments in the field of geriatrics. This preoccupation together with her earlier responsibilities in public health nursing engaged most of her adult life and are, therefore, the main substance of this work.

Sketches of Toronto's efforts toward health control in the 19th century and of the role of the tuberculosis nurse, antecedent of the public health nurse, have been included to lend historical perspective to the achievements of a new era.

Not having known Miss Dyke, with few personal letters and no diaries to draw upon, I owe a special debt to people who knew her, some of whom must not go unmentioned: Miss Florence Emory, LL.D., Miss Mary Millman and Miss Violet Carroll, all three of whom were nurses whom Miss Dyke selected as early members of her staff in the Nursing Division of the Department of Public Health. I have had advice and help, also, from Miss Eileen Cryderman, one of her later appointees, who became Director of the Division. Miss Dyke's nieces, Miss Jean West and Mrs. Catherine Barrick, filled in family background; Dr. Hastings' daughter, Mrs. Audrey Williams, told me what she remembers about her father's association with Miss Dyke; Miss Bessie Touzel, a social worker who was associated with Miss Dyke during several periods of her life, helped me place

9

her in relation to other women of her time. Mrs. Jean Good, who inherited Miss Dyke's concern for the well-being of the elderly and built upon it a distinguished career in geriatrics, has been one of my most faithful advisers, and Mrs. Doreen Nolan, now of Tucson, Arizona, cast light on Miss Dyke as a person only a few people would have recognized.

I am indebted also to Dr. Alison Prentice, Director of the Canadian Women in History Project of the Department of History and Philosophy of the Ontario Institute for Studies in Education, who has given me the privilege of association with the project, continuing into the years when this project was my chief preoccupation. Nor can I omit the unfailing assistance of the reference staff of the Institute's R.W.B. Jackson Library, especially Miss Isabelle Gibb, whose persevering pursuit of material through inter-library loans has been invaluable. Last, but by no means least, I am grateful for the encouragement and assistance of Miss Constance Gray, a public health nurse of a later day than Miss Dyke, who has read and criticised a substantial part of the manuscript and to Heather Macdougall of the University of Toronto Department of History, who checked for me the accuracy of the section on health control in Toronto in the 19th century. Most encouraging of all has been the interest and support of the Registered Nurses of Ontario Foundation. Also, I have appreciated the editorial advice and assistance of Mrs. Bernice Lever of Dundurn Press Limited.

Marion V. Royce,
Toronto, 30 April 1983.

Foreword

The work of Eunice H. Dyke, the woman who pioneered health care as first Superintendent of Public Health Nurses in the Toronto Department of Public Health, is the focus of this study. The world of medicine and nursing has seen many changes since her day, but with Dr. C.J.O. Hastings at the helm of the Department, it was a period of exciting advance in preventive medicine, and the nursing division under Miss Dyke's leadership played a uniquely creative role. The nurses, Dr. Hastings' 'life-saving crew', and those who have followed them, may be proud of their contribution to the Department and thus to the City of Toronto. It has been a flagship of public health policies and programs across Canada and beyond.

Reading the manuscript of the book, I relived my own field work as a D.P.H. student with the Toronto Department of Health in 1929. I met old friends whom I had not thought of for years. That fact is, in itself, a compliment to the research Marion Royce has done, and she has recorded the achievements of an exceptional woman. As for Miss Dyke's later years, I was led to wonder whether her pioneering experience in public health nursing may not have fostered the seed that blossomed in her forming 'The Second Mile Club' and her interest in the health and welfare of the aging population. In these preoccupations she anticipated one of the urgent social concerns of today.

Eunice Dyke was, indeed, a woman 'ahead of her time'. The book is a tribute, however, not only to her, but also to the many women who made the history of which she was a part. Moreover, it celebrates Toronto's pioneering leadership in preventive medicine and the City's care for the health and well being of its citizens.

Eva Mader Macdonald, M.D.; C.M.; D.P.H.; LL.D.; D.Hum.L.

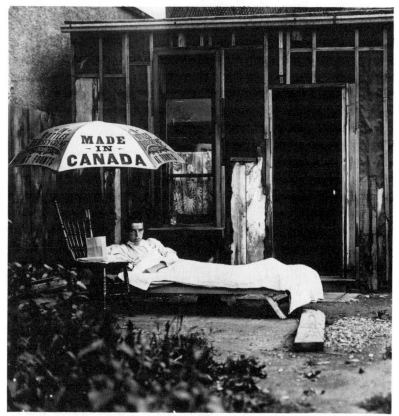

Outdoor beds for tuberculosis patients

A Prologue to Public Health Nursing

Disease Control in Nineteenth Century Toronto

Public Health is the foundation upon which rests the happiness of the people and the welfare of the state.   *Disraeli*

Disease control through government intervention has had a long history in Toronto. It began in response to the cholera epidemic of 1832. The disease had been identified in Quebec with the arrival of a ship from Limerick on 28 April. Of the 170 emigrants on board the vessel, 29 had died during the voyage.[1] That was but the beginning. Emigrants, soon numbering in the tens of thousands, continued to reach Quebec, many of them victims of the pestilence, all of them having been exposed to it, and as they dispersed westward, the sickness spread through Upper Canada. Towns along the St. Lawrence and up the Ottawa River encountered it one by one, but York, one of the largest towns, flooded with the newcomers, suffered most.[2] Its marshy ground and filth-ridden streets provided fertile seed-bed for infection. Hundreds, citizens as well as immigrants, fell ill and died, often within a single day. In the words of John Strachan (later Bishop of Toronto), the town became a general hospital. Strachan, himself, worked night and day to relieve the suffering and bury the dead. "The little town soon presented a melancholy spectacle ... the stillness of death reigned in its deserted streets, traversed continuously by cholera carts carrying the dead to the grave and the dying to the hospital."[3] Dr. Godfrey noted that some 40,000 immigrants came through York during the summer of 1832.[4]

On 20 June, a Circular issued by command of Sir John Colborne, the Lieutenant-governor, called on the magistrates of each affected district to form a board of health with

13

authority to enforce "such arrangements as a due regard to the preservation of health may require". A sum of £500 was put at the disposal of each district with the understanding that there be no unnecessary expenditures.[5] A board of health was appointed in York, but lacking legal authority to enforce its regulations, the members were unable to cope with the rapid spread of the disease among fear-stricken people. The sick, afraid of being sent to hospital, often failed to report illness until the point of death. If they went to hospital, it was to die and be buried from there. By autumn, this first epidemic had passed its peak, and in February 1833, the Circular was reissued in legal form.[6] A new board of health was appointed in York, but the onslaught of the disease had lessened, and it was not until the summer of 1834 that the next outbreak, even more serious than the first, occurred in Canada.

Meanwhile, on 6 March 1834, the Assembly had passed an Act to extend the limits of Town of York and incorporate it as the City of Toronto.[7] Elections were held later in the month, and with a majority of Reformers in the Council, William Lyon MacKenzie was appointed first mayor of the municipality. Two early measures passed by the new Council had a bearing on sanitation and public health.

The first, "An Act concerning Nuisances and the Good Government of the City", included prohibition of various 'nuisances' that were hazards to public health.[8] The second, The Public Health Act, established a Board of Health comprised of the Mayor and four Councillors to be appointed annually, with "authority to enforce the laws of the Province providing against infectious and pestilential diseases". The Act set out in detail prohibited sources of infection such as stagnant water, exposed animal carcasses, offal, unsound meat and other garbage. Suitable persons were to be authorized to examine cellars, lots, alleys, sinks or privies and remove 'all nuisances', and anyone who did not comply with the Regulations was subject to a stiff penalty.[9]

"Streets were cleaned, sewers dug, middens abolished, groggeries mitigated and mire and mud superseded by plank and McAdam", wrote Rev. C. Dade.[10] Sanitary conditions remained hazardous, however, and with the arrival of more emigrants, cholera again became epidemic. The new board of health, appointed in 1835, sought advice from the

14

Upper Canada Medical Board. This board of five physicians, appointed by the Lieutenant Governor to license individuals authorized "to practice physics, surgery and midwifery in Upper Canada", was first organized in 1818. The board recommended that public sewers be constructed to drain cellars and gutters and carry off surface water and also that the city employ scavengers who would remove animal and vegetable remains every day.[11] Nevertheless, one epidemic after another threatened the health and well being of the city. Recurrence of cholera followed further waves of immigration in 1845 and 1854, and in 1847, a virulent form of typhus brought by refugees from the potato famine in Ireland took its toll of lives. Smallpox was a continual hazard. Diphtheria was a special enemy of the young, and scarlet fever was never far behind. Repeated epidemics of typhoid were caused by contamination from the Bay and from wells poisoned by seepage from outhouses and sewers.[12]

Public health laws had been enacted by the Assembly in 1835 and 1839; the former provided for the appointment of health officers in every town in the Province with authority to carry out measures similar to those the City of York had taken upon itself,[13] and the Act of 1839 enlarged upon the earlier one.[14] Both, however, were designed for emergencies and made no provision for ongoing services, and municipalities remained indifferent to day to day problems of public health. The Public Health Act of 1849 passed by the Union Parliament gave the Governor authority to appoint a central board of health with power to issue regulations to be put into effect by local boards of health but it also was to be proclaimed only 'in certain emergencies'.[15] Moreover, although the colonial government was responsible for expenses of the central board, local authorities were accountable for costs they incurred, and they resented having to carry out the instructions of an autocratic central body.[16] Nevertheless, the 1849 statute remained the basis of public health administration in the Province until well after Confederation, and the first public health law of Ontario, passed by the Legislature in 1873, had similar limitations. The Public Health Act of 1882, however, reflected broader understanding of the need for permanent services and the involvement of the medical profession.[17] (This Act and similar legislation adopted by the other provinces of Canada were passed as a result of action of the British Parliament which had consolidated all its existing health laws in the Public Health Act of 1875.)[18] It established a provincial (central) board of health of seven members, at least four of whom must be medical practitioners, and increased the responsibilities of local boards. The central board was instructed to study vital statistics, carry out sanitary investigations and enquiries into causes of mortality in general as well as of epidemics. It was also to monitor the effect of 'localities' employments, conditions and habits and other circumstances upon the health of the people...". The findings would then be the basis of suggestions for the prevention of contagious and infectious diseases. To administer this legislation, a part-time provincial officer of health was appointed.

The Government had moved well beyond earlier conceptions of public health administration, but the central board had no authority to ensure that local boards carried out their responsibilities. This lack was corrected by the Public Health Act of 1884[19] which spelled out in detail the powers and duties of local boards and authorized municipalities of more than 4,000 inhabitants to appoint a medical officer of health and a sanitary inspector and fix their salaries. At the same time, the post of provincial officer of health was made full-time, and Dr. Peter Bryce, who had been the part-time appointee, now devoted his career to the work, continuing in office until 1904. His commitment to the health and welfare of the Province during those years earned him the title, 'father of public health'.[20] Meanwhile, the City of Toronto, without waiting for the legislation of 1884, had appointed its first professional medical officer of health on 12 March 1883. He was Dr. William Canniff, an able physician and surgeon who had had wide and varied experience.

Toronto, planning to celebrate its fiftieth anniversary, was now a budding metropolis. A lively competitor of Montreal, its historic rival, it had become an important centre of trade, commerce, and industry. Following a boom period after Confederation, however, the city had weathered years of depression, and despite the jobs being created as new industries were developed, unemployment persisted, especially among the growing numbers of immigrants for whom Toronto was a magnet. The annexing of adjoining districts had also swelled the population, and municipal services lagged behind needs. There were congested areas of badly built houses that lacked proper drainage, and many families had only well or cistern water for domestic use. Garbage and refuse collected in the streets, and raw sewage emptied in the Bay polluted the waterfront causing conditions that fostered disease.

Dr. Canniff, an ardent sanitarian, took up his duties with vigour although his role was restricted to consultation with the Markets and Health Committee which in 1877 was assigned duties for which the municipal board of health had been responsible. During his first year in office, he directed a house to house inspection of "some 17,000 premises". This first sanitary survey of the city was the basis of a comprehensive report of living conditions that Canniff submitted to the Committee with recommendations for action. When the revised Public Health Act came into force in 1884, the City Council decided at once to comply with its terms, and a Board of Health was appointed with Canniff as its Executive Officer. From that time until he resigned in 1890 because of ill-health, he strove towards his goal to make Toronto the healthiest city on the continent. At first, the authorities and the public were slow to recognize the need for sanitary reform, but Canniff, undaunted, continued to direct attention to disease-breeding conditions. Health inspectors were appointed to instruct householders "how to correct insanitary evils", and "sanitary improvement was sought by persuasion rather than coercion". Plumbers were engaged to inspect the plumbing and drains in new buildings. Water mains were laid as new streets were opened up. Proper sewers replaced open ones like Garrison Creek; in one year, 143 privy pits and most of the wells were closed. Sewage was emptied farther out into the lake, reducing pollution on the waterfront, and steps were taken toward making the Islands a healthful resort for citizens in the summer. In 1885, to prevent the spread of smallpox, centres were opened in fire halls where physicians employed by the city vaccinated all comers free of charge, and in the following year vaccination was made compulsory for children in the public schools. Responsibility for quarantine and fumigation in cases of contagious diseases was assigned to one of the health inspectors. To reduce pollution of the atmosphere, owners of large factories were directed to use smoke consumers. Dr. Canniff, however, made further recommendations that went unheeded, and in his last annual report, he challenged the city to wake up to a new day. "Toronto", he said, "is no longer a village or small city but a metropolis of goodly proportions, requiring corresponding conditions".[21]

To this day sanitation remains an urgent concern of public health administrators, but after 1890, bacteriology and therapeutic immunology (the use of serum and vaccine) became a major emphasis in their work. Public health was being revolutionized by the scientific discoveries of the three nineteenth century giants: Louis Pasteur, who evolved the germ theory and began the pasteurization of liquid foods; Joseph Lister who, recognizing the application of Pasteur's discovery to surgery, discovered antisepsis, and Robert Koch, a founder of the science of bacteriology, who discovered the germ of tuberculosis and identified the cholera bacillus. It was not by chance, therefore, that Dr. Charles Sheard, who was appointed Toronto's Medical Officer of Health in 1893, was not only a physician and surgeon but a scientist as well. He had held the Chair in Physiology and Histology in Trinity Medical School, lecturing to medical students and working with the Toronto General Hospital, where he assisted in setting up laboratories, sponsored the use of the metrotome, (a cutting instrument used in operating on the uterus, later perfected and called an hysterotome) and introduced the mounting of histological and pathological specimens. During his years as Toronto's medical health officer, he brought about sand filtration and chlorination of the city's water supply, though its effect on the death rate was not apparent until after he had resigned.[22] He coped with epidemics of diphtheria, scarlet fever, and typhoid and took steps to have hospital facilities for the treatment of tuberculosis increased. By the time he retired, the health of the city was reported to be reasonably good with sanitation improving, but in this latter aspect of his work, he encountered opposition and sometimes defeat. In 1900, when he condemned the sanitary facilities and ventilation of 16 schools that the City Council had directed him to examine, a majority of the members of the Public School Board voted against a motion to proceed with necessary improvements. They thought that the criticism suggested neglect of duty on their part, and "the discussion ended in nothing".[23]

Already in 1907, Dr. Charles Sheard, by appointing a woman as "City Tuberculosis Nurse", had introduced a pattern of work that became pre-eminent in the policy and practice of the Department of Public Health. No longer were male inspectors the only staff members of the department. Even so, public health nursing was still an untried discipline when, in 1911, his successor, Dr. C.J.O. Hastings, appointed Eunice Dyke. She became head of Toronto's public health nurses, and in long association with Dr. Hastings, built a division of public health nursing that was a model among public health services in Canada as well as further afield.

The Tuberculosis Nurse

There are many different enterprises that call the trained nurse into action, and none more important than instructing and nursing tuberculosis patients in their homes, where poverty and unsanitary conditions hold sway.[25]

In the early years of the twentieth century, tuberculosis, the Great White Plague of the North, challenged the skill and ingenuity of physicians in all parts of the world. Substantial progress in the treatment of the disease had been made since Koch's discovery of the tubercle bacillus in 1882, but it was still the cause of a fifth of all deaths. Sanatorium treatment that provided rest, fresh air, sunshine and suitable nutrition was accepted as the most effective means of coping with the disease, always provided there had been early diagnosis.[26] But at the turn of the century there was only one sanatorium in all of Canada, the Muskoka Cottage Hospital, which had been opened in 1897.[27] Dread of infection as well as inadequate provision for treatment prevented other hospitals from admitting tuberculosis patients.

While the disease was no respecter of persons or social class, it was the poor among its victims who caused most alarm. Shunned like lepers, their only refuge in Toronto was the House of Providence, a charitable institution that had been founded in 1856 by the Sisters of St. Joseph, "to succor the rejected of the community".[28] Consumptives were accepted there without distinction of creed and cared for until death and burial, but many victims of the disease were left without care. Then in 1901, under pressure from the City Council, the general hospitals began to set aside wards for tuberculosis patients, and by November, Dr. Sheard reported that both the Toronto General and St. Michael's Hospitals had done so. Meanwhile, the Western Hospital had agreed to provide accommodation for 30 patients inside 10 days, if $1,200 were raised to erect tent wards for them. Interviews conducted by reporters of *The Evening News* found public opinion favourable to the idea, and one respondent hoped that "a public consumptive sanatorium would be erected soon".[29] In fact, a second hospital to the north, the Muskoka Free Hospital, began to admit patients in 1902, and the Toronto Hospital for Tuberculosis opened its doors in Weston in 1904.[30]

Already, however, new ways of coping with the disease were being tried. For more than a decade Dr. William Osler, since 1889 Physician-in-Chief of the Johns Hopkins Hospital in Baltimore, had urged home treatment of tuberculosis patients.[31] He believed that, if patients had a better understanding of the disease and carried out hygienic directions given by a competent physician, many deaths might be prevented, and contagion substantially lessened. In that year, in order to examine the hospital's experience with victims of the disease, he called for volunteers from among the senior medical students who, under his supervision, would visit outpatients in their homes. The students' task would be to get to know the patients and other members of their families and, being careful not to antagonize them, take note of the environment in general. They were to explain to the patient the nature of the disease, why contagion occurred and how to prevent it. Most important was to make clear the necessity of destroying the sputum that contained the germs of the disease for, if not carefully disposed of, it would infect others. They were instructed also to stress the curative effects of sunshine and fresh air and suggest ways of ensuring these in home surroundings.

Two women students responded to Dr. Osler's call and once a month throughout a twelvemonth period reported their findings to him. Then in the autumn of 1900, at the first meeting of 'The Laennec', a society that he had organized for study of tuberculosis, one of the students reported

20

on the domestic and social conditions of 190 victims of pulmonary tuberculosis in the Baltimore area who had been visited regularly. The work of these two young women had demonstrated how conditions that fostered tuberculosis might be alleviated, and shortly Dr. Osler was enabled, through a special fund, to appoint a nurse to carry on the service they had begun. So it was that in November 1903, Reba Thelin, a member of that year's class of the Johns Hopkins Training School for Nurses, became the first 'tuberculosis nurse'.[32] The Osler project, a prototype in the crusade against tuberculosis, had opened "a new sphere of usefulness to the trained nurse".[33]

This new occupation in preventive medicine and public health pre-supposed the usual subordinate relationship of nurse to physician, but the 'tuberculosis nurse', entrusted with carrying out the treatment prescribed by the physician, had considerable scope for independent activity. To quote Dr. Theodore Sachs, "The mere outline of a consumptive's regime is much easier than its execution". The nurse's ingenuity and her understanding of the patient determined the effectiveness of the treatment. She was, therefore, considered to be much more nearly an equal partner of the physician than was the case in other branches of nursing.

Meanwhile in Toronto, as in large American cities, the incidence of tuberculosis had grown at an alarming rate. In 1906, it was the cause of 445 deaths in a population of 253,720.[34] So the Trustees of the Toronto General Hospital, on the advice of Dr. Alexander McPhedran, doubtless inspired by Dr. Osler's example, decided to establish a tuberculosis outpatient clinic that would cooperate with the sanatoria in efforts to halt spread of the disease. When Dr. Harold Parsons was asked to assume supervision of the clinic, however, he refused unless he might have the assistance of a visiting 'tuberculosis nurse'. Alas, the projected budget made no provision for a nurse, but Mrs. P.C. Larkin offered to underwrite the salary and other expenses for a limited period. Christina Mitchell, an 1888 graduate of the Hospital, was appointed to the post and became the first tuberculosis nurse in Toronto.[35]

Miss Mitchell was an outstanding nurse who, having worked in the nursing service of the New York City Mission, was fully aware of the nature of the responsibilities entrusted to her. The chest clinic of the Hospital which she attended once a week was the point from which she set out to visit patients in their homes in all parts of the city.

Several visiting nursing services under private auspices were already well established in Toronto. There was the Victorian Order of Nurses, founded by Lady Aberdeen in 1898, which supplied nurses trained in hospital and district nursing to care for the sick who were unable to obtain the services of a qualified nurse in their homes. Also, for a still longer time, nurses of the City Mission and the Toronto Nursing Mission, who were dedicated to "the alleviation of human suffering and spiritual necessity", had visited the homes of the poor, irrespective of creed, and often given the sick bedside care. Deaconesses of the Anglican, Methodist and Presbyterian Churches, whose training included a unit on elementary medicine, were similarly "quick to respond to every call for help". Miss Mitchell won the cooperation of the women of all these services and made clear to them her role in caring for tuberculosis patients from the Hospital Clinic as distinct from the more general nursing care they offered. Nor did she overlook charitable organizations in the community such as the YMCA, the YWCA and neighbourhood missions of the churches as important allies of the tuberculosis nurse.[36]

Although Miss Mitchell remained in the position for only one year, she left the service well established. Her immediate successor, Ella Jardine, was followed after three months by Elizabeth (Lilly) Lindsay, a Toronto General Hospital graduate of 1905. By the summer of 1907, the Larkin Fund had been used up, and Dr. Parsons turned to Dr. Sheard with a request that a tuberculosis nurse be employed by the city to work in cooperation with the hospital.[37] On 7 July 1907, the City Council, on Dr. Sheard's recommendation, endorsed this plan which was to cost $600 a year.[38] Forthwith Miss Lindsay was transferred to the staff of the Department of Health and became the first 'city nurse' in Toronto's history. The only change in her work pattern was that she was required to report twice weekly to the Medical Officer of Health.

Miss Lindsay resigned in October and was replaced by Janet Nielson, who came to be a strategic figure in public health nursing in the city. A Toronto General Hospital grad-

22

uate of 1897, she had been a night supervisor in the hospital and had spent several years also as Head Nurse in the Toronto Free Hospital for Consumptives. Her title in the new post was "City Tuberculosis Visiting Nurse", and her area of work included both the city and its outskirts. When she began there were 23 patients in her roster. Most of them were patients of the clinic, but some were reported from other sources, although doctors were not yet required to report tuberculosis patients who were in private care. In addition to home visits, Miss Neilson assisted in the Tuesday tuberculosis clinics at the Hospital and, as from April 1908, in a second weekly clinic on Fridays. About the conditions of work at this time Eunice Dyke later wrote:

> It is interesting to note that nursing cases were the rule and that night nursing was not uncommon, also that car tickets for the nurse, and relief, including nursing supplies, eggs and milk, were provided from a fund placed at the disposal of the General Hospital. The car tickets were discontinued in about six months with a recommendation to the nurse that she try to get them from the city. This arrangement she was unable to effect.[39]

Not only was the work exacting, but also a growing number of requests for care added to the nurse's responsibilities. In 1907 St. Michael's Hospital opened a clinic for diseases of the lungs,[40] and although it was not possible for Miss Neilson to assist in another clinic, she did accept requests for home visits to patients from other sources. In 1908 the National Sanatorium Association (N.S.A.) appointed a visiting nurse to work with patients who were being admitted to or discharged from the sanatoria at Weston and Muskoka.[41] She resigned in 1910, however, and the service was discontinued until, in December 1911, the N.S.A. opened a Free Dispensary that held clinics on Tuesday and Friday afternoons and evenings with a visiting nurse, Julia Stewart, as its 'motor force'.[42] The close collaboration of this N.S.A. service with the Department of Health and the hospitals added greatly to the effectiveness of the crusade against tuberculosis in Toronto.

The Heather Club, organized in 1909, through the initiative of seven nurses who were graduates of the Hospital for Sick Children, was another ally in the crusade. For a long time these nurses had been concerned about babies and young children who had been exposed to a family member with tuberculosis. Day after day, with their tired, anxious mothers, they were crowded together in the waiting room of the Hospital's chest clinic. From time to time, the clinic physicians and nurses collected funds among themselves to provide necessities for the health of the children, but there was need of more reliable assistance. The seven nurses consulted Dr. George Porter, Secretary of the Canadian Association for the Prevention of Tuberculosis, about what should be done and, as a result, formed the Heather Club, a name they chose because it suggested "fresh air on wind-blown hills of heather". The motto of the Club was *'Prevention Rather than Cure'*, and its aims and objects were threefold: (i) to aid anti-tuberculosis work with children 14 years of age and under; (ii) to give instruction in the care of patients and how to prevent spread of the disease to members of the family, and (iii) to provide suitable nourishment, clothing and corrective materials that parents could not afford. For many years Heather Club members continued to assist in the care of 'contact cases' among children, helping countless families and working closely with the public health nurses.[43]

Already in this early period, it was recognized that expansion of the city nursing service had become essential, if the crusade against tuberculosis in Toronto were to succeed.[44]

A New Era in Public Health

The year 1910 was crucial in the development of public health services in Toronto. It had become apparent that public concern should encompass not only sanitation and the control of communicable diseases, but also the prevention of disease and promotion of the health of the community. Dr. Charles John Oliver Hastings was a proponent of this wider concept. In June 1905, in a paper read before the Convention of the Ontario Medical Association, he had decried "the enormous rate" of infant mortality in the Province. Out of 48,642 deaths in 1903, there had been 6,700 deaths within the first year of life, and 10,162 before the age of fifteen.

24

These deaths, Dr. Hastings declared, had been "largely preventable". He believed that with resolute administration and education of the public, disease that never should have occurred could be brought under control. So he challenged members of the Association to add to their ambition to cure disease "the higher and nobler position of preventing it". Furthermore, he thought that education for prevention must come from the medical profession, but the means to accomplish it must be provided from the public purse too much of which was being spent on bringing immigrants into the country. In common with many, perhaps most, of his contemporaries in the medical profession, Dr. Hastings believed that, because of inadequate supervision of immigration, Canada was becoming "a dumping ground for misfits and undesirables": "whole families of degenerates" from the slums of British and European cities. This 'foreign element', it was contended, made up a high proportion of patients in insane asylums and consumptive sanatoria, and funds spent on their maintenance might better be devoted to "the health of our own people".[45]

For Dr. Hastings, however, the public health challenge was personal as well as professional. In December 1902 typhoid fever traced to impure milk had taken the life of his own small daughter and set him on a relentless crusade to arrest the appalling loss of life from preventable diseases. Already planning for early retirement when the post of Medical Officer was offered him, he nevertheless took up the task with characteristic vigour. He was well-read, knowledgeable about current developments in medicine, and, having been in private practice in Toronto for more than 20 years, was well versed in the health needs of the City. He was closely associated with the Academy of Medicine and was a member of the Senate of the University of Toronto, one of four physicians chosen to represent the University's graduates in his field.[46]

An able administrator, he saw the task before him in large perspective with, at the same time, an awareness of essential detail. Tall, handsome, kind and courageous, blest with imagination and a sense of humour as well as "a great fund of common sense", he also possessed "a dominating personality". He won many a victory over a Board of Control that gasped at his demands for increased health services. If, as sometimes happened, he was obliged to accept defeat, he never failed to warn the Board that there would be deaths that might have been prevented.[47] Occasionally, he went further. There is a story, perhaps apocryphal, certainly typical, of the funeral of a child who had died of diphtheria shortly after a proposal to expand the immunization program had been thwarted. A commanding figure with a fine head of iron grey hair, he towered over the mourning relatives and heard the clergyman intone: "The Lord giveth, the Lord taketh away. Blessed be the name of the Lord." Then, through the awed silence, came Dr. Hastings' voice, loud and clear, as he paraphrased the familiar words, "The Lord giveth, the community taketh away. Cursed be the community."[48]

He considered public health a challenge with social and economic, as well as medical dimensions. Epidemics resulted from poverty with its comcomitants of poor housing and inadequate nutrition. "Even the great white plague is not merely a human disease. It is a social disorder."[49] Individual diagnosis and treatment alone could not effect a lasting cure. Diagnosis and rehabilitation of the family, the social unit to which the patient belonged, were equally essential. The economics of the health question led him to think that a system of health insurance would be "a measure of extraordinary value", an opinion that he developed in an address before the Canadian Medical Association in June 1917.[50] The Department of Health, when he took over, was small and insignificant, "concerned with sanitation and the control, rather than the prevention, of epidemics". In the course of his 19 years of leadership, it gained world-wide recognition as an instrument for the prevention of epidemics and the promotion of public health.[51]

Dr. Hastings wasted no time on preliminaries. Only a few days after assuming his new post, he undertook to convince the Board of Health that a bacteriological and chemical laboratory for the analysis of water, milk and 'all kinds' of food was an immediate necessity. He believed that the efficiency of the Department's work would 'hinge' on the quality of a laboratory service under competent scientific direction to rival any others in existence. "The work done in the laboratory must be such as to defy adverse criticism of any Board of Health on the continent," he declared. His candidate for the directorship was Dr. G.G. Nasmith, at the time, Associate Director of the Laboratory of the Provincial Board of Health, whose services, he had "reason to believe", could be obtained if prompt action were taken. Dr. Nasmith was a bacteriologist and biological chemist, who, during the previous eight years, had done "valuable work, dealing with water supplies, milk supplies, and sewage disposal of large cities, and ... all measures dealing with the prevention of disease and the spread of contagion". He was a man of high academic attainment whose laboratory experience added to his university training had "so disciplined his mind" that he could grapple with even the most complex problems of public health. The estimated cost of the project would be between $3,000 and $3,500, and Dr. Hastings assured the Board that, with such equipment, the Toronto Department of Health "need not fear the criticism of any similar laboratory ..." He had captured the imagination of the Board members. They recommended that funds up to the amount of $4,000 be requested and that Dr. Nasmith be appointed Director of the Laboratory, at a salary of $3,000 per annum. On 24 October, the City Council approved the recommendation and instructed the Medical Health Officer to prepare the needed specifications and the Board of Control to advertise as soon as possible for tenders for the work.[52]

In the following year, Dr. Hastings obtained another concession from the Board of Control, this time, a grant of $800 to investigate slum conditions in Toronto. His report, dated 5 July 1911, described the situation as "quite as bad as in European and American cities but fortunately thus far limited". The worst conditions existed in the Central District where recent immigrants were living in a density of 82 persons to the acre. "There is a rear-tenement under the morning shadow of the City Hall occupied by six families", he wrote. In the other five districts investigated, density of population was lower, but there were houses unfit for habitation, unsanitary privy pits, no drainage, inadequate water supply, overcrowding and exhorbitant rents. Quoting Sydney Webb, he described the situation:

Soul-destroying conditions of one-roomed dwellings which make decent life impossible, ... absence of proper light, air and privacy, leading to physical and mental suffering and

27

inefficiency, ... and he added that such conditions "must not be permitted in Toronto". The slum dwellers were not there by choice; furthermore they had welcomed the Board of Health inspectors.[53]

"Prompt action is needed", he told the Board of Health, and he set forth steps to be taken to arouse public concern and work out ways of coping with the mounting problems. "We require a good housing by-law with provision for adequate enforcement, suburb garden cities with rapid transportation, and a proper scheme of city planning". Among all Dr. Hastings' concerns, however, community education in public health was pre-eminent. The entire community must be involved, and education was the instrument to that end: "We must so enlighten the public as to the control of diseases that they will demand that if they are preventable they be prevented ... We must reach every man, woman and child from presidents and chancellors of our universities to emigrants who cannot read".[54] Cooperation and education were, in his view, the twin foundation stones of public health administration. All divisions of the Department of Health must work together and cooperate with all other departments of City Government as well as with hospitals, schools, citizens' organizations and social welfare agencies in the community.

Nor were the children of the city overlooked, as witness the "Swat the Fly Campaign", a veritable children's crusade, that Dr. Hastings fostered in the summer of 1912. *The Star* offered prizes ranging in value from $1.00 to $25.00 to a total of $200.00 and dramatized 'the tournament' daily with catchy slogans about 'man's pest'. Competitors were boys and girls under the age of 16. At specified times, the flies were counted by measuring the quantity in the bottle containers in the office of the Medical Officer of Health, who was judge of the contest. Filling bottles with other materials to increase the bulk disqualified a competitor, and anyone resorting to the breeding of flies was liable to prosecution. At the end of six weeks, 3,367,680 flies (21,048 ounces) had been destroyed. Beatrice White, a girl of 14 or 15, who had 'swatted' half a million flies, was winner in the competition.[55] "Oh yes" recalls his daughter, a woman in her seventies, "Father had me swatting flies along with all the other children in Toronto". In this way Toronto's children, like those of Mao Tse-tung's China almost four decades later, learned that flies are carriers of germs and that to get rid of them would help to keep the community free from disease.

Dr. Hastings was confident, also, of the efficacy of the written word and, shortly after assuming office, he launched a monthly *Health Bulletin*, its mast-head reading, "Sanitary Instruction is more important than Sanitary Legislation". Including information from all branches of the Department of Health, the bulletin was distributed through the schools in order to reach families and was sent as well to all relevant institutions and organizations. Isabel Creighton Wilson is one of many who remember the health bulletin and how their parents, especially mothers, heeded the information it brought into their homes from month to month.

The educational task that Dr. Hastings envisaged, however, required more than publicity and fly-swatting crusades. At its centre there must be a corps of public health nurses who would visit the sick in their homes and, through "heart to heart talk", instruct and advise about the care of the patient and other members of the family. The nurses would ascertain the social conditions of the home and whether the family income was sufficient to ensure adequate nutrition. They would also see that 'contact cases' were taken to a clinic. He believed that women had "wonderful natural advantages" for this role in preventive medicine and that nurses, with knowledge and discipline gained from years of training, had "an accumulation of assets" that uniquely fitted them for the life of service that was needed.[56] Furthermore, he realized that, if the incidence of tuberculosis were to be reduced, the visits of public health nurses must not be limited to clinic patients, and from early in 1911, physicians were required to notify the Department of Health of all cases of tuberculosis in their care. Then it became necessary to appoint an additional nurse in order to ensure that all victims of the disease were adequately cared for.

The nurse selected to fill this post was Eunice Henrietta Dyke whose appointment was announced in the *Health Bulletin* for May 1911:

The Health Department has been fortunate in securing Miss Eunice Dyke, a graduate of Johns Hopkins Hospital, to take charge of the Tuberculosis work of the Department. With her will be associated Miss Janet Neilson, who has already done much good work in Toronto. Miss Neilson will for a time continue to act as Dispensary Nurse for the Tuberculosis clinic of the Toronto General Hospital. Miss Dyke will act in the same capacity at St. Michael's Hospital. Every case of Tuberculosis and every tuberculosis house of which information can be obtained is being indexed and filed for reference in order that we may be of the greatest possible assistance to the community by education and looking after cases that need our assistance.

As Toronto's public health services were developed and extended under Dr. Hastings' leadership, Eunice Dyke was entrusted with growing responsibilities. Both were strong personalities, and they by no means always agreed. Miss Dyke accepted the authoritative role of the physician, however, and, throughout her life, retained nostalgic memories of the time when Dr. Hastings and she worked together in mutual respect.

Chapter One

Eunice Henrietta Dyke

The evolution of public health nursing in the past quarter century is a social phenomenon of first importance.[1]

When Eunice Dyke took up her new post in the Department of Health in May 1911, she was a tall, beautiful young woman of twenty-eight with unmistakable personal dynamism. Having been prepared for her profession at the Johns Hopkins Training School for Nurses, she was committed to public health nursing and aware of the role of the tuberculosis nurse. Furthermore, her period of training had been interrupted by a year spent as a patient in the Muskoka Sanatorium, an experience that gave her personal knowledge of the disease that she hoped to help cure. After graduating in 1909, she remained in Baltimore for a short time doing private nursing and then returned home to care for her Aunt Tilly (Matilda Ryrie Smith) who was terminally ill with cancer at her home in Orillia. After her aunt's death in September 1910, she again took up private nursing, and in the following year, when Dr. Hastings decided to add another nurse to his staff, she was recommended for the post by Dr. Nasmith, who had recently been appointed Director of Laboratories.

Eunice was the fifth of six children of Samuel Allerthorn Dyke and Jennie Ryrie. Samuel, a son of Thomas Jefferson Dyke and Jane Allerthorn, was born in Lockport, New York, in 1845. The Dykes claimed descent from one, Anthony Dyke, who though "not a dissenter", sailed for America on the 'Pilgrim ship' *Anne* in 1623. His descendants were all United States citizens, but the Allerthorns, emigrants from Yorkshire, were unable to adjust to life in

31

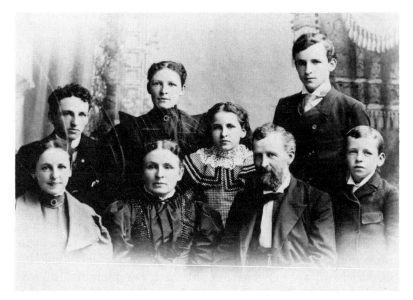

The Dyke Family — circa 1894

Back row: James Ethelbert, Jennie Ethel, Eunice Henrietta, Samuel Allerthorn
Front row: Margaret Winnifred, Jennie, Samuel, Frederick Gordon

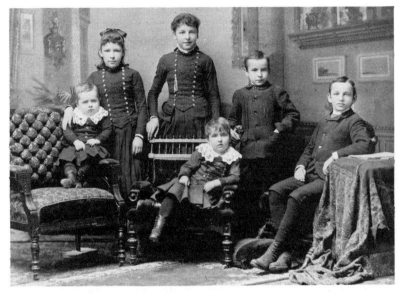

The Ryrie Family — circa 1864

(after Daniel's death)

Back row: Elizabeth, Jennie, William, James
Front row: Harry, Matilda

the new republic, and in 1829 Jane's father, John Allerthorn, took up land in a settlement of United Empire Loyalists in the Niagara Peninsula. Nine years later, Jane eloped with Thomas whose business in transport by ships on Lake Ontario and the Erie Canal and later by railway, kept him in touch with both sides of the international border. Samuel, their fifth child, grew up in Canada at Dundas where as a young man he opened a drygoods store. However, responsive to religious influence, he decided to enter the Baptist ministry and went to England for two years of study at Spurgeon's College in London. Prior to his departure, visiting the Bond Street Baptist Church (later Jarvis Street Church) in Toronto, he met the lovely Jennie Ryrie who sang in the choir. The story (perhaps apocryphal) goes that he winked at Jennie, and after the service she accosted him gaily: "Come back when you're ready to be married." This he did and they were married in June 1871, he was 26, she 21.

Jennie was the eldest of three daughters of James Ryrie and Margaret Piggott. James, who was a watchmaker, came from Caithness in the highlands of Scotland, while Margaret was the daughter of a Scottish schoolmaster who settled with his family in Three Rivers, Quebec. There James and Margaret were married, and in 1849, with their infant son Daniel, they moved to Toronto, where Jennie was born in the following year. Two daughters, Elizabeth and Matilda, and three sons, James, William and Harry, completed the family. On 1 July 1867, Daniel (Dan) who had just graduated from the University of Toronto, gold medallist of his year, was drowned off Centre Island in the Toronto Bay. William, the middle son of the other three, entered the business world as a travelling salesman, while James and Harry learned their father's craft of watchmaking, and in 1882 established the firm, Ryrie Brothers Limited, Watchmakers, Jewellers and Diamond Merchants. Already in 1879, a similar firm, Henry Birks Limited, had been founded in Montreal, and the two firms had frequent dealings. Then Harry Ryrie died in 1917, and in 1924 Henry Birks Limited bought out James and also purchased the Harry Ryrie Estate. The new firm was established as Ryrie-Birks on 7 April 1924 and remained so until 1947 when the name was changed to Henry Birks and Son Limited. A family tie was added to the Ryrie-Birks connection when Henry Birks' son, Gerald, and Margaret, a daughter of Harry Ryrie were married 21 August 1924.

The successful partnership of James and Harry Ryrie had brought prosperity that fostered social prestige which the relatives shared, as it were, by osmosis. The founder of the family, James Ryrie who died in 1888, was a deeply religious man, and he and his family became active members, at first, of the Bond Street Baptist Church and later, of the Jarvis Street congregation. They were interested also in the welfare of the community. It is remembered, for instance, that James, the son, left money in his will for concrete benches in Toronto parks.

When Samuel Allerthorn Dyke and Jennie Ryrie were married, Samuel was the pastor of Parliament Street Baptist Church, a recently organized mission of the Bond Street Church. His work there was 'singularly successful', and he went on to launch other congregations, including the College Street Baptist Church where he remained as pastor for two years. Later he left the pastorate to raise funds for Woodstock College, a Baptist institution in Woodstock, Ontario, at the same time visiting and organizing churches, including some in the United States. Returning to local work in 1895, he became pastor of Lansdowne Avenue Baptist Church and later moved further west to a congregation that eventually became Parkdale Baptist Church.[2]

The family lived in various parts of Toronto, holidaying at Kew Beach in the summer. By the time Eunice was in high school, however, their home had been established in the west end of the city. She passed the matriculation examinations at Parkdale Collegiate and went on to Normal School, as her two sisters had already done. Eunice specialized in kindergarten work and then taught in a private school called St. Monica that was run by a Miss Philpott at the corner of Bloor Street and Avenue Road, where the Park Plaza Hotel now stands. Mary Millman, whose small sister was a kindergartner at that time, while Mary was in a higher grade, remembered Miss Dyke as a lovely looking young woman who, of all the teachers, was most liked by the pupils.

Meanwhile, Miss Dyke's two older brothers had become established as watchmakers, and in 1898, Ethel married Joseph West. In June 1901 their mother died, and although the strong family bond that she had fostered continued, her death brought many changes to the Dykes. Their father went to the United States and became Pastor Emeritus of a Baptist Church in Melrose, Massachusetts. There he married Clara Bartlett, a member of his congregation, who left a small patrimony that his children eventually inherited.

In 1902, Winnifred married John Fox, while in August 1905 Eunice went to Baltimore to register at the Johns Hopkins Training School for Nurses. Later Gordon joined the Army and during World War I became an officer in the 48th Highlanders. After the war, he studied law and practised as a member of a law firm in Toronto until his death from cancer in June 1931. That was just a month after the death of their father. Rev. Dyke had returned in 1921 after the death of his second wife to live his last ten years with Eunice and Gordon. Previously in 1930, Ethel (Mrs. West) had died of cancer, and Eunice too, was a victim of this disease. She had three operations for cancer in 1930, 1940 and 1958.

The frequency of cancer in her family and among relatives led Miss Dyke in 1952 to seek the assistance of her cousin, Dr. Norma Ford, a geneticist, to trace the history of the disease through several generations. Norma Ford, whose married name was Walker, was the daughter of Rev. Dyke's sister, Hattie. The two women identified a sufficient number of cancer victims to justify the tentative conclusion that the disease had stemmed from the Piggott family line. Margaret Piggott, Eunice Dyke's grandmother, had died of cancer. In recent years, Mr. Frank R. Stone, a grandson of James Ryrie, has made a hobby of collecting genealogical information on the Ryrie family. He has kept records of deaths from cancer among family members up to the present that appear to confirm the result of the work of Miss Dyke and her cousin.

Eunice, who resembled her father in both facial features and temperament, was a clever child, lively, self-assertive and tenacious: characteristics that stayed with her through life. Fond of pretty clothes, as a child, she took special pride in her 'Sunday best', which, to the vexation of her mother and the horror of her sisters, she was not always willing to keep for the Sabbath. One of her nieces recalls a story of how, in defiance of her mother, she persisted in wearing her Sunday shoes to school until Mrs. Dyke declared in despair that she simply could not go on arguing with Eunice. That the family income could not encompass such 'extravagance', a fact of which her sisters were acutely aware, seems not to have occurred to Eunice. In any case, it did not deter her from having her own way. Economy in the household was Jennie Ryrie's concern. Her husband ignored the problem, and, had not more affluent members of the Ryrie family frequently come to her aid, it would have been even more difficult for her to make ends meet.

Although Samuel Dyke showed little concern for family finances, he was the figure of authority in the family, and Eunice grew up in an atmosphere of male domination. Throughout her life she remained convinced that the husband and father was rightful head of the household. At the same time, she appears to have inherited more than a little of her father's commanding bent. Some people who knew her in the full bloom of her career go so far as to speak of her as having been a tyrant, and there are those who confess to having felt, like her mother, that they simply could not go on arguing with Eunice. However, no one disputes her foresight and administrative capacity or her integrity. She is also described as having been unerringly correct socially. Her father's eloquence was an especial element of her heritage. People still remark about the range of her vocabulary and when she appeared on a platform, she was impressive in speech and manner as well as in appearance. "We were always proud of her," recalls one of her nurses who remembers those early days.

At the time when Miss Dyke decided to become a nurse and give her life a new direction, nursing, like teaching, was so plainly seen as an extension of the female role in the family that it was open to women without question. Moreover, Florence Nightingale's introduction of systematic training for nurses had made it an approved alternative to teaching as gainful work for young women "with a refined upbringing". In the United States, the service of nurses in the American Civil War had given it the status of a profession[4] and had influenced Canadian attitudes. By the turn of the century there were several recognized hospital nursing schools in Canada, but Eunice decided to go to the United States. "She may have wanted to get well away from home

37

and family," remarks one of her nieces. Whatever her motive, she chose one of the most famous hospital schools on the continent: The Johns Hopkins Training School for Nurses in Baltimore.

Johns Hopkins, the Quaker philanthropist, who left his great wealth for the founding of both a university and a hospital bearing his name, specified that "a training school for female nurses" should be established in connection with the hospital. He wanted to ensure competent care for the sick in the hospital wards and he also believed that a supply of well trained nurses would benefit the entire community. He had come close to death during a cholera epidemic that struck Baltimore in 1832; that experience at 29 had convinced him of the importance of skilled nursing. In that same year the disease had spread disaster in the Town of 'Muddy York'.

The hospital was opened in 1889, sixteen years after Hopkins' death, with a highly qualified staff of physicians, 'the famous four', all of whom were great teachers: Pathologist, William Welch; Surgeon-in-chief, William Halsted; Gynecologist, Howard Kelly, and Physician-in-chief, the renowned Canadian, William Osler. To find the right woman to be superintendent of nurses and principal of the training school for nurses proved to be no less demanding an undertaking than the selection of a medical faculty. The trustees consulted Florence Nightingale and her associate, Florence Lees, and visited well known hospitals in the United States, Great Britain and several countries of continental Europe. High standards had been set, and the post was a coveted one. Among many applicants, the final choice went to Isabel Hampton, an outstanding Canadian who had graduated from the Bellevue Hospital in New York and had had 21 months' nursing experience in Europe at St. Paul's House in Rome, an institution run jointly by the Church of England and the Protestant Episcopal Church of the United States. At the time of her appointment to the Johns Hopkins School, she was superintendent of the Illinois Training School of Cook County Hospital in Chicago.

Opening ceremonies of the Johns Hopkins Hospital were held 7 May 1889, and the first patient was admitted on the 15 May. From the beginning there were many candidates for admission, and students were selected with utmost care. Both Miss Hampton and her successor, Mary Adelaide Nutting,[5] also a Canadian, who had been one of the first graduates of the School, were concerned to maintain high standards of nursing education, and in 1896, the course was extended from two to three years. Hours of work on the wards had already been reduced to allow more time for study. Both women were also committed to the development of nursing services in the community, a concern that was shared by the medical faculty, especially Dr. Welch and Dr. Osler. Health teaching was early introduced in the curriculum, and arrangements made for a period of district nursing under the direction of a competent head nurse.[6]

Considering the quality and scope of nursing education offered by the Johns Hopkins School, it was little wonder that Canadian women of stature who aspired to become nurses were attracted to it. Until 1940, four Canadians, (all except Miss Hampton, graduates of the School), filled the post of Superintendent of Nursing and Principal. Other Canadians, including Christina Dick of the class of 1889, who spent 27 years as Residence Director, served in various capacities on the staff. In addition, Dr. Osler's position as Physician-in-chief of the Hospital and Professor of Medicine in the University, ensured close and cordial connections with the field medicine in Toronto. Dr. Hastings occasionally visited Baltimore for consultation with Dr. Osler and his colleagues.[7] Therefore, Eunice Dyke came to the Toronto Department of Health, with no small degree of prestige as a result of her association with so distinguished a school for nurses.

For Miss Dyke, the years she spent at Johns Hopkins were an indelible experience, which moulded her conception of the model nurse she had set out to become. Discipline was strict. The authority of the head nurse was unquestioned, and spontaneity discouraged. Miss Dyke never forgot an incident that occurred when she was a probationer. One day when she was dancing along a corridor delighting in the rustle of the starched petticoats under the floor-length skirt of her uniform, the head nurse, coming up to her unawares, remarked in a chilling voice, "Miss Dyke, that was most unseemly behaviour". It was a crushing rebuke, and Eunice took it to mean that, if one were to become a model nurse, one must not indulge one's fancy. From that time on, in her professional role, she stifled spontaneity and assumed a distant, dignified exterior, a strait-jacket that became habitual. Nonetheless, 'Johns Hopkins' gave its students a high standard of education. Miss Dyke became a faultless nurse on the hospital wards. In addition, from experience of district nursing, she glimpsed the possibilities of public health work that was still in its infancy. Carefully directed reading and study made her aware of the importance of keeping up-to-date with the principles of nursing and its underlying theory, both medical and social. Dr. Hastings was aware of the merits of the School, and when he introduced her to Toronto, it was with conviction of the advantages that her preparation at the Johns Hopkins School would have given her.

Public Health Nurse's Black Bag Contents

Nursing Supplies
- Castor oil
- Green soap
- Mouth wash
- Vaseline tube
- Thermometers: rectal and mouth
- Instruments: scissors and forceps
- Bags: absorbant cotton rectal tube and funnel
- Hand towel
- Gown
- Book
- Bichloride tablets
- Olive oil
- Alcohal
- Talcum powder
- Basin
- Safety pins
- Bandages - 1" and 2"

Literature on Tuberculosis and Child Welfare
- Care of Baby - 2
- Diet slips - 2
- Pre-natal care - 2
- City Order papers - 2
- Birth Registration cards - 2

Sanitary Supplies
- Spectum outfit
- Refills
- Handkerchiefs
- Paper bags

A list from page 317 of Miss Dyke's Brown Book

Chapter Two

A Mammoth Undertaking

Laying the Foundations of Public Health Nursing in Toronto's Department of Health

It was a pioneering effort. There were no precedents.   *Florence Emory*

Although Eunice Dyke's initial responsibilities were outlined in Dr. Hastings' announcement of her appointment, only her unstinting effort over a period of 21 years revealed the dimensions of the task to which she had committed herself. "The driving force behind all her work was a desire to develop a municipal public health nursing service of the highest order," says Florence Emory, "it was a worthy concept, a mammoth undertaking".[1]

She began by taking over work with tubercular patients and their families in the area from Yonge Street to Spadina Avenue south of College Street as well as responsibilities related to the chest clinic of St. Michael's Hospital. Compulsory notification of tuberculosis cases had met little opposition and by June 1912, 200 physicians had registered their cases in contrast to three just a year earlier. The number of patients to be cared for had increased proportionately: "Nearly 800 cases have been reported in writing, no duplicates being included in that number," wrote Miss Dyke. Already she was supervising the increased staff of nurses who needed initiation into a type of work in which most of them had little or no previous experience.

Equipped with their small black bags, nurses visited all positive and suspected cases, "unless the physician-in-charge stated that the services of city nurses were unnecessary". The purpose of these home visits, like those under Dr. Osler's supervision in Baltimore, was to help the family carry out the physician's instructions for patient care and prevention of the spread of infection to other members of the household. "The family of the tuberculosis patient becomes the charge of the public health nurse, and all available medical, institutional and social services are called upon to prevent the development of new cases in that family . . . . Careful instructions in all details of the daily life are reiterated and nursing care is given or secured if necessary," wrote Miss Dyke. If there were school children in the family, their names were registered with the Medical Inspection Department of the Public Schools, at that time administered by the Board of Education. In May 1913, the Board opened summer 'forest schools' in High Park and Victoria Park for children who had been exposed to the disease in the west and east ends of the city.

From the beginning, there were two voluntary organizations on whose members the Department of Health nurses depended. The Heather Club of nurses, who were alumnae of the Hospital for Sick Children, continued to carry on anti-tuberculosis work among children 14 years and under who were patients of the Hospital's chest clinic, and in 1912, the Samaritan Club was organized to assist families of tuberculosis patients from Toronto who were receiving medical care in sanatoria. The Department of Health nurses were in touch with these families but had no funds for relief and often turned to the Samaritan Club for needed clothing and additional nourishment. The Club also paid for dental and optical treatment and assisted with rent payments when the head of the house was in a sanatorium. For single men discharged from sanatoria, it provided housing until they could find work.[2]

When a patient was removed from the home, whatever the reason, the nurses arranged for fumigation and followed through to ensure that it was carried out satisfactorily. For families in need of material help they sought the cooperation of charitable organizations. Few of these were as well organized as the Samaritan Club, and the city often provided such necessities as tents or beds, suitable clothing or even railway fare to a sanitorium. Sputum boxes and paper handkerchiefs were distributed gratis as were pillows if needed, but to supply food, fuel or rent-money was beyond the authority of city nurses. Responsibility was by no means limited to 'charity' patients, however. By May 1913, fifty-five per cent of the 'private' cases in the city were also being reported, and the number was steadily increasing which in Miss Dyke's opinion was the result of "a growing public sentiment that regards the public health nurse as a public servant rather than a charity agent".

Meanwhile, contacts outside the Department were being provided for the nurses as Dr. Hastings believed that these would broaden the outlook of the staff he had begun to build. Already, in September 1911, Minutes of the 12th Canadian Conference on Charities and Corrections record the attendance of 'Miss E.H. Dyke and Miss J. Neilson' at a session on tuberculosis when Dr. J.H. Holbrook, Superintendent of the Mountain Sanitorium in Hamilton, spoke on "The Fight Against Tuberculosis". One can imagine the uneasiness of the two young women; neither of them took part in the discussion led by Dr. George D. Porter, Secretary of the Canadian Association for the Prevention of Tuberculosis. Nevertheless, the speaker's description of tuberculosis as "pre-eminently a disease of the poor" would have borne out their experience of visiting clinic patients in their homes.

Attendance at that Conference was but a beginning. In 1912 and again in 1915, Miss Dyke attended conferences on charities and corrections in the United States. In 1913 she went to Ottawa for the Convention of the Association for the Prevention of Tuberculosis and at the request of the Superintendent of School Nurses, the Board of Health authorized her attendance at the Convention of National Organizations for Public Health Nursing in Atlantic City. Also that year took her to Washington for meetings having to do with hygiene and demography and the prevention of infant mortality, the latter trip authorized by the City Council in November. Nor were such privileges reserved for her; in September 1913, two child welfare nurses were delegated to attend the International Congress of Child Hygiene in Buffalo. In 1914 there was less travel, but Miss Dyke went to Halifax for meetings of the Canadian Tuberculosis Association and the Canadian National Association of Trained Nurses.

After the outbreak of war on 4 August 1914, restraints

on spending together with growing demands for public health nursing at home, curtailed such experiences. Moreover, trained nurses were responding to calls for service with the Red Cross and the Army in Britain and in the War Zone, and new staff members had to be inducted to replace the several 'city nurses' who went overseas.

At home, in addition to their 'field' duties, the nurses were required to write daily reports of their work to be filed in the office at the City Hall, a task that was demanding but essential, for their reports formed the warp and woof of the developing service. Administration of the program was a mounting responsibility. In addition to planning for needed services and the supervision of staff, it required cooperation with medical and social agencies in the community as well as with patients and their families and, increasingly, with other departments of city government. Most exacting, however, was the search for suitable staff. While appointments were made by the Medical Officer of Health and confirmed by the City Council, they were based on Miss Dyke's recommendations.[3] Nursing education of the day included no training in public health, nor was there public recognition of need for it. Therefore, Miss Dyke set out to find "nurses with a thorough knowledge of nursing practice and health laws and high ideals of service".[4] As the work developed the education of public health nurses became one of her largest preoccupations, a concern in which she had the unflinching support of Dr. Hastings.

Her responsibilities were exacting and uncharted and there were times when she found them intimidating. In August 1911, the third month of her new position, the appointment of Christina MacLennan, the third nurse on the staff, awakened misgivings in Miss Dyke's mind about her own qualifications, and she recorded that consideration was being given to the appointment of Miss MacLennan as "superintendent of city nurses". Miss MacLennan had been supervisor of visiting nurses at the famous Henry Street Settlement in New York, experience very pertinent to conditions in Toronto. Although there is no evidence that Dr. Hastings had changed his mind about Miss Dyke filling the post, she continued to mull over the matter and over a year later attempted to explain why Miss MacLennan would not have been a suitable head:

44

any added responsibility of work resulted in lack of poise and small difficulties seemed great to her. Her work in homes had been good and her advice in record-keeping was valuable, though critical rather than constructive ... Finally, when Miss MacLennan sent Christian Science healers into two homes and adopted the philosophy herself, it was decided to allow her to take a complete rest, and she left on the 19th of March, 1912.

Returning to the subject still later, Miss Dyke noted that Miss MacLennan, after resting until autumn, had taken charge of the West End Creche where she remained until the spring of 1915. During that time, despite having to cope with "a difficult conservatism", she had brought the creche to "the front rank" and helped to bring about reforms in the Central Committee of Day Nurseries. She also established good rapport with city nurses who visited the creche daily and made follow-up visits to the homes of the infants. The record goes on, "while her work was unusual and she was very happy in it, friction developed with the Board. This may have been primarily due to Miss MacLennan's morbid sensitiveness ...". Then Miss Dyke's sense of fairness took over and she added that the difficulties might have been attributable "to the fact that the Board had been accustomed to dealing with a matron who was an upper servant rather than a highly trained co-worker".

Miss Dyke's reaction in this instance was foretaste of similar conduct in future years. That she was an astute judge of character is evident in her selection of candidates for her staff, but if her self-worth were threatened, even for no apparent reason, she had a way of cutting people down to size, and seldom, if ever, did she apologize to the person in question. Absorbed in the demands of daily life, she would dismiss the matter, but it was a tendency that undermined relationships not only with her nurses but also often with other colleagues, friends, and members of her family.

Notwithstanding personal doubts and disturbing thoughts, with guidance from Dr. Hastings Miss Dyke pressed on. Clearly tuberculosis was not the only obstacle to health in Toronto. There was an even more alarming rate of infant mortality: 150 per 1,000 live births in 1910, and an average rate of 137.2 for the five-year period 1910-1914.[5] Fly-infested houses and impure milk caused epidemics of diarrhoea during hot summers, and when autumn came infants "died like flies", said Dr. Florence Emory. At all times of the year, poverty drove many women out of their homes to work, and they were unable to nurse their babies. It was estimated that 90 per cent of those who died in summer months were bottle-fed. Improper feeding fostered debilitating disease. "Most of those who in infancy are regarded as physically unfit were healthy at birth and merely victims of bad environment, improper feeding and neglect, in short, conditions which it is possible to remove," wrote Enid Forsythe, one of Miss Dyke's nurses.[6]

Despite this optimism, there were always problems of poverty and destitution. Medical fees were costly, and physicians were seldom consulted, usually too late. The new laboratory in the Department of Health was testing both water and milk, and drastic action was taken to rid the city of infected milk. In May 1913, sanitary inspectors poured some 900 gallons of milk into the sewers.[7] Pasteurization was made obligatory in 1914, but meanwhile the pasteurization plant of the Hospital for Sick Children was the only source of pure milk for infant formulas. Civic action to alleviate the loss of young life was urgent.

In the summer of 1912, just a year after Miss Dyke's appointment, the Board of Control authorized the first measure of child welfare under municipal auspices by confirming the appointment of three nurses to instruct mothers in infant feeding. These, like the tuberculosis nurses, were under her supervision, but they were not the only child welfare nurses in the city at that time. Daily baby clinics with a nurse assisting were being held at the Hospital for Sick Children, and the clinic nurse kept in touch with the mothers to help carry out the physician's instructions. Also, several agencies conducted milk depots for the distribution of certified milk from the pasteurization plant of the Hospital, and from these depots follow-up work was done. In June the University Settlement, which already had a milk depot, established a weekly clinic with a physician and a nurse in charge. The Earlscourt Methodist Church also employed an infant welfare nurse, while the Evangelia Settlement nurse and various groups of visiting nurses included infant work among their duties. Evangelia Settlement, founded in 1907; University of Toronto Settlement opened in 1910; Central

Neighbourhood House in 1911, all were in the central part of the city. The Riverdale Settlement was in the east end.

These other infant welfare nurses joined the 'city nurses' in a conference to plan the summer's work. The Home Economics Association, which had pioneered in securing pure milk for babies, opened two additional milk depots for the summer months, and another voluntary organization made ice available. In November the University Settlement nurse was made a member of the city staff, and at about the same time Memorial Institute, a Baptist institution, began a baby clinic, the city having been invited to take charge of the nursing. Each of the agencies appointed its own physician and conducted its own milk depot, but cooperation avoided duplication. In October the Women's Dispensary in Seaton Street opened a milk depot and a baby clinic, and in 1913 St. Christopher House, Central Neighbourhood House, and the Riverdale Settlement, took similar action. The Hospital for Sick Children had agreed to supply certified milk in formula to milk depots cooperating with the Department of Public Health.

Additional child welfare nurses were appointed to the city staff for the summer 1913, and, in September, six of them were retained. Further appointments were made in November and again in January 1914. Gradually, the various clinics and milk depots were coordinated under the Department of Public Health, their nurses having been transferred to the city pay-roll. Thus the nucleus of a comprehensive program of child welfare nursing services was brought into being. On the wall of Miss Dyke's office a map of the city, with routing tacks that indicated where infant deaths occurred, provided a key to areas where intensive work was needed.

During the summer of 1913 a group of physicians interested in medical care for infants discussed the formation of a baby clinic association, but Dr. Hastings insisted that, to ensure acceptable standards in the work of the clinics, there should be close cooperation with the Hospital for Sick Children.[8] As a result, the child welfare clinics became an outgrowth of the Hospital's medical service.

The 'Brown Book', like an old-fashioned ledger in a box in the Toronto City Archives, contains Miss Dyke's record of her early years as Superintendent of Public Health Nurses

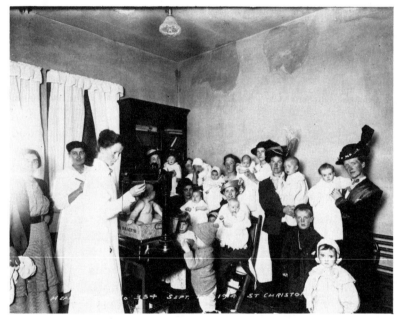

*St. Christopher's House — Baby Clinic, 30 September 1914 —
located behind Toronto Western Hospital*

in the Toronto Department of Health. In addition to her description of the work for which she was responsible, it includes information about the background of each nurse. When Miss Dyke was absent, whoever replaced her made the entries. After 1916-17, this type of recording was abandoned probably because of expanding responsibilities, but the 'Brown Book' remains a treasured resource of the history of one of Toronto's notable achievements in the pioneering days of public health nursing services. In a report written at the end of 1913, Miss Dyke described the development of public health nursing in Toronto thus far as "a history of adaptation to the work of independent agencies":

... These essential forces existed and the Department decided to correlate and stimulate rather than duplicate them. This work has been carried on by imperceptible change and to some extent unconsciously.

"Miss Dyke was keen on cooperation with other civic services," recalls Florence Emory.

Nevertheless, it was clear that all was not well. "Two groups of equally trained nurses, with two filing systems, reporting to one office and one superintendent of nurses ... seemed poor administration," wrote Miss Dyke. The nurses were having to spend too much time and money on street cars, often visiting the same homes and working with the same social agencies. Moreover, they were serving very large areas of the city and coping with such varied needs that to work through one central office was no longer feasible. In January 1914, therefore, three district offices were opened, each in charge of a supervisory nurse with oversight of public health in her district while being ultimately responsible to Miss Dyke. Then, in the following month, the Division of Public Health Nurses (later called Division of Public Health Nursing) was created to unify the administration of tuberculosis and child welfare services. Moreover, this new structure established what came to be known as the generalized plan of nursing, in that each district nurse was responsible for both tuberculosis nursing and infant care. "We decided to specialize in homes rather than diseases and to safeguard the interest of the medical specialist by office organization rather than multiplication of health visitors."

diverse agencies to secure constructive work
in the homes. The co-operation has
been sympathetic and 1912 and 1913
showed phenomenal growth in the
co-ordination of isolated social forces.
The Case Conferences were a concrete
expression of this spirit of co-operation.
At the close of 1913, over sixty agencies
held membership in the three conferences
and further conferences were contemplated.

The Public Health nurses believe
that the unit in health work is the
family — one family frequently
presenting many medical and social
problems. They believe that the nurses
of the Department of Public Health should
be qualified to assume responsibility for
the health of the homes, to carry on
educational work in the homes and to
call in specialized agents for special
needs — medical or social. With this
in view plans were being formulated
at the close of 1913, to combine the
Tuberculosis and Child Welfare groups of
nurses into one group of Public Health
nurses and to secure the additional
training required to make them efficient
assistants not only of medical but also
of social agencies.

1911 1912 — 1913 Jan 1914

Eunice H. Dyke R.N.

The Brown Book, *Miss Dyke's personal record, page 372*

Now, instead of all the city nurses working out from and reporting to the central office in the City Hall, a district office became their base. Each nurse was assigned to a particular area within a sub-district and reported to the district superintendent. Patient records were kept in the central office where they were filed under the direction of a nurse who was stationed there. Also based on the central office were two 'special directors', (later called supervisors) one for child welfare, the other for tuberculosis. The former attended the Outpatient Clinic of the Hospital for Sick Children and received physicians' orders which were delivered to the nurses in the field through her district superintendent. The field nurses' reports of home conditions, which would influence recommendations for treatment, were then transferred to the physician concerned. In other words, it was a two-way process. The special directors for tuberculosis, working with hospital clinics concerned with that disease, followed a similar routine. Calls for service received by the central office were organized by districts and delivered to district offices to be passed on to the appropriate field nurse. The district superintendent was responsible for all clinics in her district while the 'special directors' saw that consistent standards and procedures were maintained throughout the city.[9]

Neighbourhood needs that the nurse in the field could not meet were referred through her district superintendent to the central office, but every effort was made to avoid having details of district matters turned over to the central office. This system helped to strengthen cooperation with local agencies, and a growing number of field nurses acquired capacity for administration so that their work became the backbone of the service. The new organization also relieved Miss Dyke of miscellaneous details and freed her to plan for the future in consultation with the Medical Officer of Health. Yet it did not diminish her watchfulness of the entire enterprise. Surviving members of her staff still comment on her total command of the work of the Division.

However, concern for efficient administration never hindered imaginative efforts to combat infant mortality. In the summer of 1914 the Toronto Ferry Company lent the Department of Public Health one of its boats three afternoons a week from 9 July to 21 August to make possible an outing for mothers with children under two years old who were referred from well-baby clinics by the public health nurses. "It is hoped to counteract by this means the unhealthy atmosphere of the congested districts from which these children are taken, thereby lowering the death rate...., and those in charge of the undertaking report that the results have proved beneficial," wrote the Toronto Correspondent of *The Labour Gazette*.[10] Mothers responded eagerly. In a total of 19 trips, 1,963 mothers with 2,318 babies enjoyed the boatrides with a public health nurse on board to make up the feedings for bottle-fed babies, funds for supplies having been furnished by *The News*, a daily newspaper. Describing the project in his Annual Report for 1914, Dr. Hastings told the Board of Health: "Many mothers walked quite long distances, some two or three miles, often carrying their babies in their arms rather than miss the sail". The greatest value of the experiment was as an advertisement for the clinics, but it was not repeated because the results, gratifying though they were, did not justify the amount of work involved.

From the beginning, Miss Dyke shared with Dr. Hastings a conviction that the family was the essential unit of the work of the public health nurse, and families in which the mother was a wage-earner outside the home were her particular concern. Accepting the established view of the middle class of the time, she regarded such families as 'strikingly abnormal' and since they could be reached only through the day nurseries where their children were placed, arrangements to keep in touch with the nurseries took on high priority. In cooperation with the West End, Victoria and River Street nurseries, a plan that had been devised by Christina MacLennan and her Board was adopted. When a woman applied for work, her name was given to the supervisory nurse of the district and was reported to the nursery. The family was visited by a social service worker and the home placed under the supervision of the field nurse who filed a duplicate report. Either before or after receiving the report of home conditions, the nursery superintendent decided whether to accept the children.

Not all of Miss Dyke's nurses, however, were happy about such invasion of family life. As early as June 1913, Dorothy Farncombe, a graduate from the Toronto General

Hospital, who had been appointed as a children's tuberculosis nurse in October 1911, resigned to do private nursing. "She frankly stated that the aggressive policy of the nurses' work was disagreeable to her," wrote Miss Dyke, who attributed Miss Farncombe's attitude to "the terrible nerve strain of trying home conditions which made her crave simple tasks". Two years later it was recorded in the Brown Book that the Department had twice tried and failed to persuade Dorothy Farncombe to return, and someone had added: "It is possible that with a different Superintendent she might return and do excellent work."

June 1914 also saw the formation of a division of child hygiene with a filing system to record the birth of every child in the city as soon as it was registered by the physician in the city clerk's office. Current literature on the hygiene of infancy and care of the infant was sent to the mother of every new-born child with an invitation to attend the well-baby clinic nearest her home, if her child were not in the care of a private physician.

Previously, to take a well baby to a physician, let alone a clinic, had been unheard of, but gradually the practice came to be accepted as a preventive measure and a means of observing the child's growth and development.

Reporting these various developments to the Board of Health in January 1915, Dr. Hastings listed the components of the Division of Public Health Nurses: the Superintendent of Nurses, the Director of Social Service, the Medical Director of the Division of Child Hygiene, and 37 public health nurses. By this time, also, there were five district offices with a public health medical officer related to each. Dr. Hastings explained that Miss Dyke, as Superintendent of Nurses, had oversight of the entire staff of city nurses, irrespective of the division to which any nurse might be attached, and she was directly responsible to him as Medical Officer of Health. Thus Miss Dyke's status was assured.

In the beginning, the nurses had full charge of the well-baby clinics, but in 1915, Dr. Hastings persuaded Dr. Alan Brown, Canada's first trained pediatrician, a staff member of the Hospital for Sick Children and from 1919, its physician-in-chief, to accept appointment as Medical Director of a Division of Child Hygiene (later called the Division of

Child Welfare) with his salary to be paid by the Department of Public Health. It was an appointment that strengthened the link already established between the work of the baby clinics and the Hospital for Sick Children. Dr. Brown undertook the planning of child welfare work for the entire city, including the assigning of physicians to the various clinics and the organizing of their schedules. The executive work of the clinics he left to the nurse supervisor of child welfare, at that time Nora Moore, who reported to him daily at the hospital.[11] Dr. Brown profoundly influenced the outlook and practice of Miss Dyke and her nurses in the fields of child health and welfare. Like Dr. Hastings, a lifelong advocate of preventive medicine, he believed that infant mortality was one of the great social and economic problems of the nation. "The baby is the citizen of the future," he wrote, "and his [sic] rights we cannot afford to neglect."[12] He adhered strictly to the rule not to send a child home from hospital until he received the nurse's report of home conditions upon which he depended in recommending treatment.

As the work of the Division developed, Miss Dyke became increasingly convinced that it could never be truly effective without more meaningful cooperation among social work agencies. In exasperation, she wrote, "the lack of organization of the social forces of the city has been a menace to public health". So, with Dr. Hastings' backing, she tackled the problem by working with social agencies through 'case conferences' which had begun to meet periodically in various parts of the city.[13] These conferences, which Miss Dyke described as a concrete expression of cooperation, coordinated otherwise isolated social forces and became the nucleus of the Neighborhood Workers' Association (N.W.A.). Representatives of the four existing conferences met at the City Hall on 22 January 1914 and appointed a committee to draw up a constitution that would provide for a central organization. A month later a mass meeting, also held in the City Hall, adopted a constitution for an association of churches and social organizations "to organize family work in Toronto" and to be "the vehicle through which gifts of service or money by organizations or private individuals may be effectively applied".[14] The city was divided into nine districts and three secretaries who were to be responsible to Central Council of the N.W.A. were appointed, their salaries to be paid by the city through the Social Service Commission, a group of five businessmen interested in philanthropy. It was a confusing arrangement for the secretaries because the Commission, as the body paying the salaries, tended to assume command of their services. By 1917 the N.W.A. Council took steps, therefore, to set up the Association "on its own basis".[15] The N.W.A. was the precursor of the Family Service Bureau of Metropolitan Toronto.

Dr. Hastings believed that there was an inevitable social work component in the role of his public health nurses. Reporting to the Board of Health in November 1914, he emphasized their "unlimited possibilities in an educative and instructive way, both as regards disease, vice and crime", and he continued: "The routine duties of the public health nurse unconsciously make a social worker of her, for when she is looking after the sick members of the household, she is also considering the income of the home, the nutrition of the family, and general sanitary conditions. The family is to her a social institution, and with a knowledge of the fact that ignorance and poverty is [sic] responsible for most of our preventable diseases, she appreciates . . . that social diagnosis is sometimes even more important than medical. With our nurses in possession of a good working knowledge of social service work, one visit to a home can do what two, three, or four have been doing in the past."

Then came his final flourish: "It must be apparent that a well organized Division of Public Health Nursing is a very valuable asset to every Department of Public Health".

It was an exposition that might justify a steadily increasing staff of public health nurses, at the same time reflecting current thinking of the public health movement that conditions which prevent disease are the conditions that maintain health. Moreover, it underlined the reason for an appointment that had been made a year earlier. In the autumn of 1913, Arthur Burnett, a Methodist minister trained in social work and aware of social conditions in Toronto, (with Miss Dyke's concurrence, if not at her suggestion,) was appointed to the staff of the Division of Public Health Nurses. He was to develop the social work of the Department of Public Health in relation to other civic and voluntary agencies and assist in training the nurses of the

Department in social service aspects of their work. Burnett was an Englishman from Bristol who, in the summer of 1909, had taken part in a survey of social conditions in Toronto made by students of Victoria College. Having worked for several years in the Whitechapel District of London, visiting people in their homes to collect data about living conditions, he became a key individual in the Toronto project to which, as a skilful photographer, he also contributed telling pictures. As a result of the project, the Student Christian Social Union was formed, and as President of the Union in 1910 Burnett arranged a series of lectures and discussions on social questions at Victoria University in which such outstanding citizens as J.J. Kelso, who founded the Children's Aid Society in 1891, and University of Toronto President Falconer participated. Also, working with Kelso, Burnett became associated with the group that founded Central Neighbourhood House, a social settlement free from sectarian influence, which opened its doors at 84 Gerrard Street West in September 1911. Here, he lived as a student-worker during the first year of the settlement's existence and in 1912 was awarded a fellowship for study at the School of Philanthropy in New York. Having completed the one-year course, he applied for the post of head of the University Settlement in Toronto, but the appointment went to Dr. Norman Ware, who came from the University of Chicago, and Mr. Burnett, undoubtedly known to Dr. Hastings, took the post in the Department of Public Health.[16]

Both Miss Dyke and Mr. Burnett became associated with the organizing of the Neighbourhood Workers' Association, and, with Dr. Hastings' approval, Mr. Burnett accepted the secretaryship of the Central Council. In June 1914, a Division of Public Service was formed within the Department of Public Health with Mr. Burnett as its Director. The new Division, renamed a month later as the Division of Social Service, was given responsibility for assisting the public health nurses to make use of cooperative relationships that the N.W.A. initiated for them with welfare organizations. In dealing with social problems of families they visited, the nurses became field agents of the new Division and the district superintendents attended meetings of local units of the N.W.A. to report cases as directed by Mr. Burnett. These N.W.A. local units did not dispense relief;

rather each was 'a clearing house' for the needs of families in the district, and relief was provided by an appropriate social service organization or agency.[17]

This complex pattern of work was further complicated by growing antipathy between Miss Dyke and Mr. Burnett. In January Miss Dyke moved into the field of social service without reference to Mr. Burnett. Unemployment in the city during the winter of 1913-14 had brought miseries of which no one was more aware than the public health nurses. Civic action was tardy, but finally on 14 January, the Board of Control authorized a grant to open a registration bureau for the unemployed. Two days later, *The Toronto Daily Star* initiated a relief fund to fight hunger and want, the proceeds to be used to aid families of men registered at the Bureau. The public health nurses, with student volunteers enlisted by the University Settlement, spent four days assisting the Bureau to get underway and then undertook to make a survey of the need by visiting the homes of men who had registered. Where relief was needed, they referred the family to the nearest clergyman or social agency. No record was kept of the number of visits made, but Miss Dyke wrote that the nurses worked heroically. As a result the registration card of the Bureau was altered to include additional information, and individuals were referred directly to either a clergyman or a nearby social agency.

In defence of this departure from the nurses' usual routine, Miss Dyke explained that her Division had been aware of "the weaknesses and possibilities" of the exercise, but the motive of the survey was "largely to prevent misuse of the Star Fund". She acknowledged that unnecessary visits had been made but believed that the formation of three additional N.W.A. groups within a short time was "to a large extent" the result of the hurried survey which had demonstrated the city's lack of organization for constructive social work. Furthermore, *The Toronto Daily Star* had persuaded the Social Service Commission to cooperate with the Neighborhood Workers' Association.[18]

Nevertheless, despite Miss Dyke's optimism, the project appears to have been abortive. Minutes of a meeting of the Downtown Association of the N.W.A., at which both she and Arthur Burnett were present, record the appointment of a committee to draw up a scheme of outdoor relief and seek cooperation from the Social Service Commission "in furthering their plan and presenting it to the Board of Control".[19] There is, however, no evidence of connection with the January episode, although Miss Dyke seems to have thought of it as a prototype of the cooperation that was later achieved. In any case, she plainly needed to justify the exercise which must have been an irritant in her relationship with Mr. Burnett. Again, when representation of the Department of Public Health on the Central Council of the N.W.A. was being decided, a crisis arose because Mr. Burnett assumed that he should represent the entire Department, including the nurses, while Miss Dyke believed the latter role to be rightfully hers. After repeated conferences with Dr. Hastings, it was agreed that as Superintendent of Public Health Nurses, Miss Dyke should have a place on the Council comparable to that of the head of any city-wide organization. She was listed in Council Minutes, therefore, as representing the Division of Public Health Nursing while Mr. Burnett represented the Division of Social Service.

Not surprisingly, when Mr. Burnett resigned from the Department of Public Health in 1917, Miss Dyke expressed no regret at his departure. She wrote that the relation between the two divisions, public health nursing and social service, had been ill-defined, and cooperation unsatisfactory. She claimed, moreover, that Mr. Burnett had never undertaken to define relationships with the various social agencies either for himself or for the public health nurses. Miss Dyke's resentment of Mr. Burnett was shared by some others who worked with him who felt that he tended to seek reconciliation of views, often to his own advantage. On the other hand, some of her colleagues found Miss Dyke tiresomely obstinate in defence of her point of view, although most describe her as having been "ahead of her time".

Miss Dyke, always ready to cooperate with hospital services, sometimes acted impulsively. One such incident occurred in May 1915, when Dr. Gordon Gallie, newly appointed to the obstetrical service of the Toronto General Hospital, asked her for a nurse to attend his clinic and report on cases for which the Department of Public Health was responsible. Having obtained Dr. Hastings' consent, she sent in one of her nurses without having consulted either Jean Gunn, the Hospital Superintendent of Nurses, or Jane

Grant, Head of the Social Service Department of the Hospital. When the omission was brought to her attention Miss Dyke realized that it might have caused a serious breach in relationships. Happily, however, a cooperative plan was worked out in a conference with Miss Gunn, Dr. Gallie and a senior member of the Obstetrical Division of the Hospital. Henceforth, the public health nurses were to see that Jane Grant was informed about all patients they referred to the obstetrical clinic and, in turn, she would notify the Department of Public Health whether hospital or home care was needed. In her Brown Book, Miss Dyke recorded several similarly impetuous actions "because of their probable effect upon future developments". She seems to have accepted the blame for such lapses in judgment, relieving the physician of any responsibility. Moreover, she cheerfully accepted the 'red tape' involved in maintaining cooperative relationships with hospital staff.

Meanwhile, the nurses had become convinced that lack of knowledge and skill among mothers was a cause of many of the problems affecting children's health, and in October 1914, the Division of Child Hygiene changed one of its bi-weekly clinics in each of 10 locations into a class in mothercraft. Arrangements were made with the Technical School to have a teacher visit each location once in two weeks, and in alternate weeks the nurse of the clinic took charge of that phase of instruction. From this beginning, mothercraft became an integral part of the work of the clinics.

In the following year the responsibility of the Division of Public Health Nurses was extended to another area of child welfare. Since 1897, by provincial law, inspection and registration of maternity boarding houses and the protection of infants assigned to them had been entrusted to local boards of health.[20] In Toronto, a medical inspector, Dr. Harley Smith, was appointed to carry out this task for the municipality, and as a result the number of deserted infants had been reduced substantially. Not satisfied with a routine inspection, Dr. Smith undertook to weed out undesirable 'baby homes' and get rid of foster mothers who, chiefly concerned with money-making, tried to obtain more children than they could care for properly. He interested trustworthy women in child welfare and induced them to take one or more children into their homes. As the number of foster homes increased and the number of children in each was reduced, the death rate among infants decreased.[21] By 1915, however, the task had become overwhelming, and Dr. Smith asked Miss Dyke for the assistance of a public health nurse who would visit the homes and advise foster mothers about the care of infants. Mary Stirritt, a recent graduate of the Toronto General Hospital, who was completing her probation as a member of the public health nursing staff, was chosen for the new post. As the problems were complex and often the result of social conditions, it was decided that she should report to Mr. Burnett as Director of the Division of Social Service.

When Dr. Smith went overseas in 1916, the work was reorganized, and Miss Stirritt was transferred to the Division of Public Health Nurses as special supervisor of licensed foster homes. Stationed in the central office in the city hall, she had general supervision of the homes, with responsibility for issuing and renewing licenses. Inspection and visiting were done by the field nurses, each of whom might have one, two or more foster homes, sometimes none, in her district. The nurse usually visited each of them once a week, more often if the baby were ill, and advised the foster mother about care and feeding. She also arranged for medical supervision of the child in the nearest baby clinic where the infant was weighed, its progress noted, and any errors in feeding corrected. The field nurse was often able to recommend foster homes that were suitable for infant care, and she also reported those where babies were being boarded without the knowledge of the Department of Public Health.

Miss Stirritt, herself, careful not to duplicate the work of the field nurses, kept in touch with developments in each home and visited the district offices at regular intervals in order to meet the nurses and discuss their work with them individually. In addition she attended weekly conferences in the central office at which Miss Dyke met with the district superintendents and the Supervisor of Child Welfare Clinics. Reports indicate that, under this arrangement the quality of foster infant care rose steadily. In this, as in each area of public health nursing for which she was responsible, Miss Dyke's administration ensured growth and improvement of service.

Chapter Three

Fresh Challenges

As new needs for public health nursing arose in the community, Miss Dyke's responsibilities continued to expand. Typical examples of such new challenges were increasing absenteeism among civic employees and the plight of enlisted soldiers' families.

The former of these occurred first in 1914 when the Department of Public Works considered stopping the sick-pay of its employees in order to check 'malingering'. On low wages, the workers had no savings to fall back upon, and if such action were taken, Miss Dyke feared they would "sink readily into conditions of living that would create a public health problem". She saw it, moreover, as an opportunity for the public health nurses to do some constructive health teaching. Through Dr. Hastings' intervention, it was decided, therefore, that the city nurses would investigate these cases of illness and, following their usual routine, obtain medical care when necessary.[1] Shortly this service was extended to all departments of City Government, and, in 1918, accounted for 2,560 home visits, including cases of bedside nursing for civic employees under Workmen's Compensation, for which the nurses had also been made responsible. Ostensibly a public health measure, this plan doubtless commended itself to city officials as a measure of economy as well. No consideration appears to have been given, however, to causes of low morale that might have led to malingering, and the employees (unorganized workers) had no say in the matter. Nor did the nurses complain about the additional work required of them. Moreover, the action was an interesting example of the pervasive, not to say persuasive, influence of Dr. Hastings, as with the full cooperation, if not

61

outright urging, of Miss Dyke, he fostered an expanding role for the public health nurses under her direction.

The outbreak of war in August 1914 brought an even greater extension of the work of Toronto's public health nurses when the Academy of Medicine decided to provide free medical services for dependents of soldiers who had gone overseas. Col. Fotheringham went to Miss Dyke with a proposal that the Academy create districts that would conform to those of the Division of Public Health Nurses with a view to having the nurses in the field available when nursing care was needed by soldiers' families. Shortly, this voluntary work of the physicians was made a function of the Toronto and York Patriotic Fund, and Enid Forsythe, one of Miss Dyke's most able nurses, was given indefinite leave to act as Secretary of the Medical Bureau of the Fund. She worked from the central office of the Nursing Division and directed the public nurses as field agents. At the same time, Miss Forsythe was assisting with the work of the Social Service Division, and in March 1915, when the Patriotic Fund asked that she be transferred to their office to help with other aspects of their work, Dr. Hastings intervened to appoint her permanent assistant in the Division of Social Service, giving as much of her time to the Patriotic Fund as its Medical Bureau might require. In August 1915, an additional nurse was appointed to take over the Fund's work, and Miss Forsythe was released to give full-time to the growing work of the Social Service Division. Later in the year, when Dr. Hastings was asked to lend a public health nurse to assist in a health centre experiment of the Instructive Nurses' Association in Boston, Enid Forsythe was chosen for the assignment. Miss Dyke was on study leave in Boston at the time, and it is more than likely that she played a part in this arrangement, for she had full confidence in Miss Forsythe's ability. The experiment in patriotic service continued, and in the end, was felt to have had permanent value in demonstrating the possibilities of cooperation with nurses of the Victorian Order, as well as having advanced "the education of physicians in the use of the graduate nurse for obstetrical work in middle class homes". There was also hope that the experience would have helped to overcome the tendency to think of the public health nurse as a charity agent rather than as a public servant, a notion that Miss Dyke, and Dr.

Hastings greatly deplored.

Still another challenge to Miss Dyke's Division was how to offer public health care to non-English speaking new Canadians. Toronto, though still ardently British in spirit, was no longer a wholly Anglo-Saxon city. An influx of European and Asian immigrants had radically altered the ethnic composition of the population. By 1911, within a total population of close to 375,000, there were 18,000 Jewish people and over 4,000 Italians, as well as growing numbers of other Europeans, and newcomers continued to come before and after the war of 1914-1918.[2]

Restrictions on Oriental immigration limited the numbers from that part of the world, and in Toronto at the time there were just a few Japanese and slightly over a thousand Chinese. Among these latter tuberculosis was endemic, and there was a high incidence of deaths among the patients who were reported. Because cases were not reported until the disease had reached an advanced stage and often discovered only at the point of death, it was difficult to control the spread of infection. The Department of Public Health, having been informed that one patient had returned to China, was led to believe that others followed a similar pattern. However, it was feared that even before a victim of the disease left the country, the illness had become sufficiently advanced to have spread the infection. There was little the nurses could do except to try to ensure that cases were reported and thus brought within the scope of their care.

European immigrants were also ready victims of infectious diseases. Exploited by landlords whose only interest was in the collection of rents, they often lived in overcrowded, unsanitary conditions that they had no control over. The health of such families was a particular concern of the public health nurses who, bent upon "education and prevention", were, in true Toronto tradition, exclusively English-speaking. Consequently, they found "the foreigners", as they called the immigrants, suspicious of efforts to help them prevent disease.

Language being the most obvious barrier to understanding, it was decided to appoint two "language nurses". In November 1914, therefore, Matilda Simone, an Italian-speaking nurse, was appointed to work with Italian families. Though born in Rome, she had grown up in Toronto and

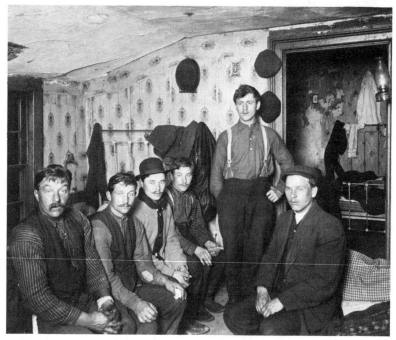

Unhealthy crowded rooming house, King Street, 1912

had trained as a nurse at St. Michael's Hospital. A year later, Zara Price, who, born in Russia and trained in St. Petersburg School of Nurses, had also had a postgraduate course in a Vancouver hospital, was added to the staff. Miss Price was an especially valuable nurse in that she spoke not only Russian, but also German, Ukrainian, Polish and Lettish. The district superintendents passed on to these two nurses the names of families with whom the other nurses were unable to communicate. Shortly, too, all literature on the care of infants distributed by the Division was translated into both Italian and Yiddish.[3] In January 1920, a third language nurse, Pareska Stamenova, was appointed to work with Macedonian immigrants whose numbers were growing, especially in the east end of the city. In addition to the usual program of instructing mothers in infant care, Miss Stamenova was to teach the mothers English.[4] By that time, the nurses of the Department of Public Health were also involved in medical inspection of schools, and there are Macedonian-Canadians today who recall how, as children, they submitted without protest to Miss Stamenova's routine examination of their teeth and eyes.[5]

Language was not the only barrier, however. Equally formidable were the fears and forebodings of the immigrant mothers. Far from their native soil, they were baffled by the nurses' unfamiliar ways of infant care. They insisted, for instance, that a child should not be bundled into layers of clothing that the mothers thought essential to its comfort. As a matter of fact, even Canadian-born mothers were often taken aback at the new-fangled ideas about dressing babies. One of these tells about Miss Dyke visiting her on a hot midsummer day in 1928, when her son was four weeks old. To the mother's dismay, as Miss Dyke held the child, she took off one garment after another leaving him in diapers only. Then giving him back to his mother she remarked, "Now your baby will be more comfortable". "And," recalls the mother, "he was". However, so radical a departure from traditional ways was less acceptable to perplexed immigrant mothers who misunderstood and often resented the nurse's interference even if the infant might be more comfortable.

In short, the nurses, even those who spoke one's language, were outsiders in an immigrant community. Nevertheless, they were there, calling and to be called in case of need, and over the years mutual respect often blossomed in friendship.[6]

When the tuberculosis and child welfare nursing services were combined to form the Division of Public Health Nurses, Miss Dyke had noted that staff rules must be formulated. Without precedent but with continuing change and development, flexibility had seemed desirable, and an association of public health nurses organized in 1913 had dealt with problems as they arose. From the beginning of the service Dr. Hastings had ruled that the staff should wear street clothes rather than nurses' uniforms. Even today nurses of Toronto's Department of Public Health do not wear uniforms.

It was not until September 1915 that Miss Dyke and her assistant, Miss Moore, undertook the drafting of precise regulations relating to such matters as hours of work, salaries, leave of absence, equipment, car-fare and emergency calls. In comparison with today's salary levels, it is interesting that in 1915 a probationary nurse earned $65.00 per month, and a permanent nurse $900.00 per year.

Miss Dyke left for study leave in October, and Miss Moore, who had been appointed Acting Director in her absence, finished the task. The new rules left little room for doubt about what was expected of the Division's nurses, but they, like hospital nurses of the day, had no say in the policies that governed their conduct.

In 1917 an anomaly in Toronto's public health services was corrected, and the reorganization that followed was a triumph for Eunice Dyke. For years there had been overlapping between medical services in the schools and the work of nurses in the Department of Public Health. Dr. Hastings' predecessor, Dr. Charles Sheard, had looked upon medical services in the schools as "a pure fad instituted principally by women",[7] and in 1910, the Board of Education, bypassing the Board of Health, had introduced medical inspection in the schools. Dr. W.E. Struthers was appointed chief medical inspector of schools, and dental inspection was introduced as well. At the same time, the Board of Education brought Lena Roger, a nurse who had organized school nursing service in New York City, to pioneer a similar service in Toronto.[8] In Miss Roger's words, the objective was "to teach children how *to be* healthy and how to *stay* healthy". The

66

nurse, through visits to the homes, brought families into the program. She became a friend and counsellor to mothers and was, at the same time, an aide to principals and teachers.[9] By 1917 Toronto had 39 school nurses with a supervisor who worked from the offices of the Board of Education. The value of their work was not in dispute, but nurses from the Department of Public Health, who were responsible for communicable diseases and maternal and child welfare, were visiting many of the same homes. Mary Millman, a voluntary visitor from the Central Neighbourhood House who later trained as a nurse and joined Miss Dyke's staff, remembers times when as many as three nurses visited the same home in one day: a Board of Education nurse, one from the Department of Public Health and still another from the Victorian Order.[10]

Aware of the waste in this duplication, the City Council, in 1916, applied to the Provincial Government for legislation authorizing transfer of medical services in the schools from the Board of Education to the Board of Health. Dr. Hastings encouraged this initiative as "a means of consolidating public health work in the City of Toronto", but the two boards failed to reach an agreement, and no action was taken. Dr. Hastings persisted, however. Unlike his predecessor, he had long been an advocate of medical inspection in the schools[11] and now, at his urging, the matter was submitted to ratepayers in the Municipal Election of January 1917. The result was unequivocal. "The polls gave evidence by a large majority that the people had confidence in the wisdom of their Medical Officer of Health", wrote Miss Dyke in her 'Brown Book'. In April 1917, the change in jurisdiction was made, the necessary legislation having been passed in the meantime.

Under Miss Dyke's leadership, adjustment to the new situation occurred without delay. School nurses were given positions on the executive staff of the Division of Public Health Nurses to assist in the planning, and a large part of the work was done by district superintendents. A new district was opened in Parkdale, and small sub-districts were delineated in other districts. The nurses now had to spend less time in transit and became better acquainted with the areas where they worked. Transfer of part-time medical officers of the Board of Education to full-time posts in the Department of Health made available badly needed resources to care for emergency cases and for patients who were unable to pay doctors' fees. Moreover, since dental services were included in the transfer, it had become possible to provide dental treatment for pre-school children. Also in September, nursing services, previously restricted to public schools, were extended to the separate schools.

"Re-organization was soon in running order", wrote Miss Dyke. The 'generalized' pattern of work adopted when the Division was decentralized in 1914 was extended to include school nursing. Henceforth each city nurse carried out all the public health nursing services in the sub-district to which she was assigned. Only bedside nursing was omitted. Her role in public health nursing was comparable to that of the general practitioner in medicine. She did not replace the specialist in medicine or in social work but saw that their skills, if needed, were drawn upon, and she continued health teaching with the patient and his or her family. Her main support came from regular consultations with colleagues and with the district superintendent to whom she reported. Policies were agreed upon in regular conferences of the district superintendents and the supervisors of each branch of public health nursing at which either Miss Dyke or the Assistant Director presided. Further, each supervisor had the added responsibility of maintaining relationships with community agencies concerned with her special field. Thus the 'generalized plan' not only reduced administrative costs for the city, but enabled the Department of Public Health to keep in touch with relevant developments in the community as a whole. It was one of Eunice Dyke's most valuable contributions to the public health nursing services of the city and brought her recognition throughout Canada and abroad.[12]

Meanwhile, the field of mental health presented a fresh challenge to Miss Dyke. One of the services inherited from the Board of Education grew out of preoccupation with the isolation of the 'feeble-minded' to prevent "the so-called dangers of racial pollution" that it was believed would result from their propagation. One of the promoters of this theory was Dr. Helen MacMurchy who conducted a census of the feeble-minded in Ontario in 1908 and proposed the introduction of a variety of services including special classes for backward pupils in the schools.[13] In response to this suggestion, the Toronto Board of Education had taken steps to organize some special classes and, in December 1912, decided that one of the staff of doctors "should be qualified to report on mentally defective and backward pupils".[14] Clarence M. Hincks was the one of the doctors to be given this responsibility and, having become interested in intelligence tests, he introduced them as a means of identifying pupils to be assigned to special classes. Actually, a psychiatrist, Dr. Hincks was associated with Dr. C.K. Clarke, in establishing clinical services for the feeble-minded in the Toronto General Hospital in 1914. Also, between 1914 and 1918, he and Dr. Clarke "made a survey of criminal court cases: and found 862 children with an I.Q. between 50 and 70; 818 between 25 and 49, and 114 with less than 25.[15] These findings, based on contemporary tests that were later repudiated by both men, ignored the effect of environmental circumstances and cultural background on a child's perception. They were, however, accepted as confirming a theory that identified criminality with so-called feeble-mindedness. When the school medical services were transferred to the Department of Public Health, Dr. Hincks was retained as consulting psychiatrist until 1919, when he was succeeded by Dr. Eric Clarke, a son of C.K. Clarke, who had just graduated. The public health nurses, in cooperation with the teachers, selected pupils who were backward or who caused trouble in the classroom, and the psychiatrist was responsible for testing them. Miss Dyke saw that one of her nurses, Emma de V. Clarke, a daughter of C.K. Clarke was awarded a Rockefeller Fellowship and had leave to study psychiatric nursing at Smith College, Northampton, Massachusetts, to prepare her for supervision of the mental health activities of the nurses. Miss Dyke, following Dr. Hastings' lead, was convinced that this 'mental hygiene' function of the Department was essential to maintain and build "a fitter race of Canadians", and it must involve the public health nurses.

None of the foregoing challenges matched the emergency created by the 'flu epidemic of 1918. It led to a crisis that tested the mettle of the Department of Public Health and made extraordinary demands on its nurses. Returning Canadian soldiers brought the disease with them from the battlefields of France where they had been exposed to its devastation. The medical profession in both Europe and America were caught in a dilemma, knowing neither the cause of the outbreak nor how to prevent its spread. Through his contacts with public health agencies in the United States, Dr. Hastings kept in touch with the most effective means of coping with the disease, as he and Miss Dyke went into action. Nurses were added to the staff on an emergency basis, and, with the help of the Red Cross Society, volunteers were enrolled and assigned to district offices. Nurses and volunteers worked day and night in hospital wards, and additional accommodation was opened in the Arlington Hotel.[16] Still there were not enough hospital beds, and many patients had to remain in their homes. Harrowing stories were told of households stricken to the last member without help of any kind. Public health nurses provided as much hourly nursing as possible, but many of them fell victims of the disease, and the Division was understaffed. Visiting nursing services of the city were taxed to the limit, and teachers who had escaped illness acted as clerical assistants. Dr. Hastings reported that, in October alone, 17,108 influenza visits were made. There had been 150,000 cases in Toronto, and 1,750 people had died. "The epidemic lasted approximately two months and was an unforgettable experience for all of us," recorded Miss Dyke.

Nor was the city nurses' responsibility for influenza patients limited to Toronto. Four of them, with scarcely a moment's notice, were enlisted to accompany convalescent soldiers from Red Cross hospitals at the ports of Halifax and Saint John to points across the country near their homes. In 1975, one of these nurses, Violet Carroll, recalled her bewilderment when Miss Dyke telephoned her one Sunday afternoon to ask whether she would like to travel across Canada by C.P.R. At first she thought it was a hoax, for occasionally one of the nurses, imitating Miss Dyke's voice and manner, would call a colleague and ask her to do some outrageous thing. In a few minutes, however, she realized that it *was* Miss Dyke, who had just received a message from Mrs. Adelaide Plumptre, an officer of the Red Cross Society, asking whether some of the public health nurses might be available for such a mission. If Miss Carroll were willing, she must report to the Union Station at eight o'clock that evening. Miss Dyke, always ready to accept a new challenge in situations of evident need, expected her nurses to do the same. Miss Carroll accepted the task as did the other three. Even earlier, in December 1917, when Halifax was rocked by an explosion in the harbour, 20 of the city's nurses had been sent to help care for the many victims of the disaster.[17] Not without reason Dr. Hastings called the nurses of the Department his 'life-saving crew'.

The general economic depression that followed the war years came to a head in the autumn of 1920. In Toronto, with an estimated 25,000 out of work, distress and suffering were widespread. As winter approached the air of desperation that pervaded the city was exacerbated by the frustration and resentment of returned soldiers unable to find jobs. 'A workless army' organized by the Grand Army of United Veterans marched on Queen's Park. They refused to sing the National Anthem and demanded immediate action, "deeds not words". On 11 December 1920, *The Globe* reported also, that a deputation sent to Ottawa with a request for assistance was told by Prime Minister Meighen that unemployment was "not a Federal matter". According to the British North America Act, local relief was a problem 'primarily' for municipal authorities and "in second place" for provincial governments. Moreover, conditions were equally serious in other cities, and any assistance from the Dominion Government would have to be on a national basis with no grants to particular municipalities. Shortly, however, it became apparent that the need was beyond the resources of local authorities even with any assistance that might be forthcoming from provincial governments, and the federal government accepted responsibility for "one-third of any money expended for the relief of workers unable to obtain work and in necessitous circumstances".[18]

Meanwhile, on 9 December, the City Council held a public meeting to consider the growing problems of unemployment in Toronto, and on the following morning a special meeting of the Board of Control voted a sum of $50,000 for emergency relief to be administered by the Medical Officer of Health and the Commissioner of Property. Robert E. Mills, since 1917, Director of Statistics and Social Service in the Department of Public Health,[19] was appointed executive officer to distribute the funds, and once more Dr. Hastings' 'life-saving crew' of public health nurses was called

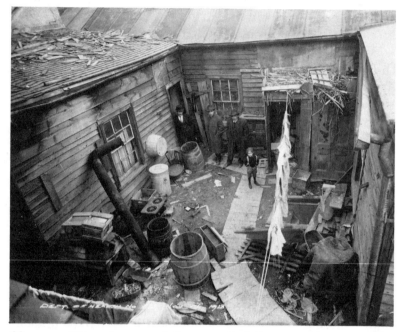

Slum conditions increased the spread of disease, 1913

upon, this time to carry on the relief work for families of unemployed men. Dr. Hastings later reported that planning was begun immediately on Saturday, 11 December 1920 and by Tuesday, everything was ready. The new organization concentrated on emergency unemployment relief, with Nora Moore in charge of a division of families, the field work being done by the other nurses through their district offices. One of the greatest problems was to coordinate emergency relief with the work of social agencies, and Dr. Hastings asked for assistance from N.W.A., which by this time included within its membership 187 social agencies. In response to the request, a worker from the N.W.A. was placed in each of the district offices of the Department of Public Health.[20] This arrangement created a closer link between the Department of Public Health and the Neighbourhood Workers' Association and was so mutually satisfactory that it was continued long into the future. It gave N.W.A. staff direct knowledge of district problems and resources, while, for the public health nurses, it provided unhampered access to the skills of social case workers. The work of the nurses had to do with the health of the community, teaching people the precepts of good health and encouraging them to do the healthy thing. If poverty or some other social problems prevented patients from carrying out their suggestions, the nurses must see that the appropriate social agency was called upon to deal with that phase of the problem, a service for which they depended on the N.W.A. secretaries. In the past, cooperation had often not been attempted because it was so difficult to achieve. The new relationship meant, also, that the nurse was freed to concentrate on aspects of health work that required her special training. Moreover, the N.W.A. secretaries became "part of the community life in a way that would have been impossible had they still worked from an office in a central place downtown".[21] It was the kind of cooperation between public health nurses and social workers that Miss Dyke believed in and worked for throughout her life.

This closer cooperation between the N.W.A. and the Division of Public Health Nursing greatly facilitated the development of hospital social service, later called hospital health service. It was one of the most highly valued programs of the Department of Public Health, in which the nurses were transferred to the Division of Social Service to organize 'follow-up work' with patients in the wards and out-patient departments of Western and St. Michael's hospitals. Shortly, the service was extended to other hospitals, and by 1918, as an administrative unit within the Division of Public Health Nursing, it employed 12 nurses who worked with all but one of the large hospitals of the city as the Toronto General Hospital had its own social service department.

Nurses assigned to the program were responsible for its several aspects: creating for patients and their families a link between the hospital and outside agencies that could provide needed medical or social treatment; gathering information about social conditions that affected individual patients for physicians and nurses on hospital staffs; advising patients on hospital wards or members of their families about health care and explaining physicians' orders to them, as well as helping patients on release from hospital to cope with difficulties of mental adjustment to illness and social problems that illness created for them.

Robert E. Mills described this 'Toronto Plan' of hospital social service as "parallel to that of a modern army". He compared the district superintendents of the Division of Public Health Nursing to "company commanders, line officer in charge of personnel", and the special supervisors as "staff officers in charge of special functions". The superintendent of hospital social services had a unique position in that, as well as being "a line and staff officer", she was responsible for personnel in one group and function in another. She had a staff of her own working in the hospitals and also supervised the hospital social service activities of the field nurses who were in continuing touch with patients in their homes. Further, she was responsible for the training of both groups in the hospital social service phase of their work. General supervision of this service, as of other functions of the Division, was Miss Dyke's responsibility in her role as Director, and she, of course, reported to Dr. Hastings.

People out of work and in need of 'city relief' had led to substantial increase in the welfare responsibilities of the Department of Public Health[23] and, in order to cope more adequately with the additional work, a welfare branch was set up in the Department in 1921. Robert Mills was appointed Director of the new branch, and Ethel Dodds its Chief Welfare Officer. Miss Dodds had had experience in social service work in Montreal and Vancouver and was well known to the public health nurses of Toronto, having been in charge of the University Settlement for 15 months and, for four years, Head Worker of St. Christopher House. The staff also included four social workers, three for family welfare and one as children's worker.[24] For city patients in hospital wards Toronto's per capita allowance was $1.50 a day, and for outpatient service the city paid 32 cents per visit. In 1921 the amount paid to hospitals was $602,203 for in-patients and $55,776 for outpatients.[25] The public health nurses had a close association with the new branch because of their responsibility for 'city patients' on hospital wards and in

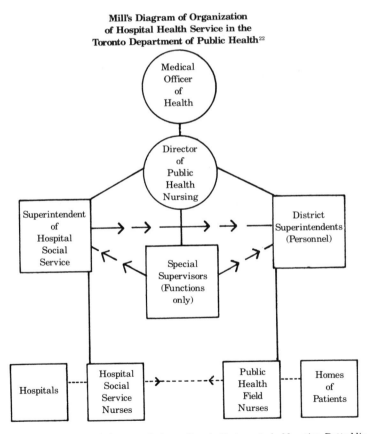

Mill's Diagram of Organization of Hospital Health Service in the Toronto Department of Public Health[22]

Solid lines indicate control of personnel. Arrow lines indicate control of function. Dotted lines indicate channel of communication between hospital and home.

outpatient clinics as well as follow-up work with all of them, including those from the Toronto General. In addition, it was the office of the public health nurses in the city hall that granted 'city orders' for hospital treatment that were authorized by the 'relief officer'. The nurses also kept in touch with homes of patients if help or advice were needed in the care of patients. In Miss Dodds, Miss Dyke found a competent and cooperative colleague with whom she enjoyed renewing contact when both were no longer in the Department of Public Health.

At the end of 1921, a decade after Miss Dyke's appointment, Dr. Hastings reported to the Board of Health that Toronto had just had the healthiest year in its history. The mortality rate had been the lowest on record, an achievement that he attributed to the work of the public health nurses. For Miss Dyke herself, one of the most gratifying developments during this period was the widening relationships of the Division of Public Health Nursing with other divisions of the Department and also its outreach in cooperation with health and welfare agencies in various fields of specialty of the supervisory nurses. In fact, the work of the Division had been restructured to meet the expanding and changing needs efficiently and effectively, clear evidence of Miss Dyke's genius for administration. For instance, the responsibilities of the Supervisor of Child Hygiene were extended to include cooperation with agencies within the Department and representation of the Director of Public Health Nursing on the Child Welfare Council of Toronto and the Canadian Council on Child Welfare. Moreover, supervisors of other special fields had similar wide-reaching responsibilities.

There had been a change, however, in the supervision of tuberculosis work. District superintendents were by now able to handle most of the supervisory duties in that specialty, but there were responsibilities in the control of disease that could not be left to them, and since the superintendent of hospital social service, worked constantly with sanitoria and chest clinics, supervision of the tuberculosis work of the Division was placed in her hands. She became the Division's representative with the Canadian Association for Prevention of Tuberculosis and with social agencies connected with tuberculosis clinics. She worked closely with district superintendents, however, informing them promptly of sputum reports, admissions to sanitoria and deaths of tuberculosis patients.[26]

Even as Dr. Hastings took pride in the achievements of the nurses of his department, however, he deplored "the regrettable lack of knowledge of their activities" in the community, and he was ever ready to explain and defend them. One of his favourite tributes to the Division of Public Health Nursing, which he cited frequently, had come from the Chairman of a Government Commission on Medical Education in Ontario, before which he and Miss Dyke gave evidence on standards in public health nursing in February 1917. Members of the Commission had gone to New York to obtain information about public health nursing, but when it was learned that they came from Toronto, they were advised to return home, "inasmuch as Toronto was leading the continent in public health nursing, and other cities were watching with intense interest the valuable work being done there". When Dr. Hastings reported this incident to the Board of Health, he added that almost every week one or more visitors came to Toronto to study methods of public health work. Moreover, during the preceding four years, 28 of the city's public health nurses had gone to posts of responsibility in other municipalities.[27] Needless to say, it was a record of accomplishment and widening influence that was equally gratifying to Eunice Dyke and convincing evidence of her administrative skills. It was now a decade since she had joined the Department of Public Health, and she had never failed to perceive new needs and to cope creatively with new challenges.

TO BE HEALTH EXPERT IN FRENCH METROPOLIS

Miss Eunice Dyke Receives Handsome Offer From Paris

At the invitation of the Red Cross League of France, Miss Eunice Dyke, Director of Public Health Nursing, will spend four months in Paris as consultant on public health nursing. The League will pay her travelling expenses and $300 a month. She will be in Paris from February to May.

Dr. C. J. O. Hastings, M.O.H., has authorized Miss Dyke to accept the position, and the Board of Health at its meeting yesterday afternoon granted her leave of absence. When the matter was brought before the board Ald. Small, the Chairman, warmly complimented Miss Dyke on the appointment.

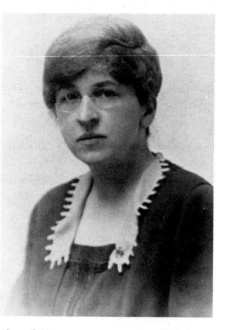

Miss Dyke's achievements are rewarded, The Globe, *14 December 1923*

Chapter Four

An International Figure

To Be Health Expert in French Metropolis Miss Eunice Dyke receives handsome offer from Paris

This headline from *The Globe*, Toronto, 14 December 1923, made Miss Dyke an international figure overnight. She had been invited by the League of Red Cross Societies to spend four months as a consultant on public health nursing, working with the League's headquarters in Paris. *The Globe* announced further that the League would pay her travelling expenses plus $300.00 a month, and she would be in Paris from February through May, 1924. The news item stated:

> Dr. C.J.O. Hastings, M.O.H., has authorized Miss Dyke to accept the position, and the Board of Health at its meeting yesterday afternoon granted her leave of absence. When the matter was brought before the Board, Ald. Small, the Chairman, warmly complimented Miss Dyke on the appointment.

Ironically, however, there was no mention of the Canadian Red Cross Society, the Canadian affiliate of the League which had been organized in 1919 to provide means of communication with other national Red Cross societies and to coordinate relief work. In 1863, when the International Committee of the Red Cross was formed by a group of Geneva citizens with delegates from 14 countries, its purpose was foreseen as the care of the sick and wounded of armies at war and the victims of disaster. After the First World War, however, the Treaty of Versailles envisaged a

79

broader role for the movement. National Red Cross societies were invited to undertake work in peace-time for "the improvement of health, the prevention of disease and the mitigation of suffering", and the League of Red Cross Societies was brought into being to correlate the work of national societies in carrying out the new mandate.[1] A headquarters was set up in Paris and various technical departments established, among them a nursing bureau that was to be the focus of Miss Dyke's work on the League's behalf. This assignment, a high point in her career, had the added glamour of a first visit to continental Europe and also to England, where she was to spend a month in the service of the League. Miss Dyke's salary in 1924 had been $1,600. She was given leave without pay but after her return she received one month's pay to compensate for extra travel costs.

One evening after her return, wearing a beige silk gown in the tubular fashion of the day with a russet coloured velvet evening cloak, both of which she had bought in Paris, she described for her nurses the experience of those four months. There is no record of her talk, and her surviving nurses have forgotten what she said. They remember her, however, as an imposing figure in her Parisian gown, and there was magic in the idea of travel abroad with highlights from France and England. There is no clue to where she lived in Paris, but the League's offices were in 'la rue Velasquez', near 'Parc Monceau', one of the loveliest parks in the city, and even the hard pavements of Paris would not have deterred her from exploring the shops, gardens and museums that to this day enchant visitors to that historic city.

In London, housing had been arranged for her at the Cowdray Club in Cavendish Square, and the usual two-week period of residence had been extended for the month of her visit. The Cowdray Club, named for the Viscountess Cowdray, who had contributed generously to its founding, had been opened in 1922 as a women's social club associated with the Royal College of Nursing but its membership was not confined to members of the College. Other nurses and women from other professions might belong, while "women who did not follow a profession as a means of livelihood, were also admitted". There was only one restriction, no one under 18 or past 70 was eligible for election to membership. The house, which had been the home of the Asquiths[2] for several years, was famous for its broad staircase. There were pleasant reception rooms, a spacious dining-room, and more than 50 bedrooms that had both central heating as well as hot and cold running water, unusual amenities in England at that time.[3] In a letter to Dr. Hastings, Miss Dyke wrote that it was her "first experience of a club of that kind", and she had enjoyed living there. Miss Dyke had lived in the Toronto Graduate Nurses' Club for one year, but it was modest, even crude, in comparison with the Cowdray Club.

She also told Dr. Hastings that she had visited the House of Commons and seen Westminster by moonlight when she was the guest of honour at a dinner party given by the Matron of St. Thomas's Hospital. 'Observation visits' to the chief London hospitals had absorbed the greater part of her time, but she had attended several meetings, including a conference of hospital matrons held in Leicester. That was one of the only two journeys she made outside Greater London, the other to Bradford in the West Riding of Yorkshire. While in London she gave a series of lectures and led discussions in the League's International Course for Nurses at Bedford College of the University of London. This she found a rewarding experience as she was impressed by the calibre of the students, most of whom were from countries of Continental Europe.

However, problems as well as pleasures marked those four months. In the same letter to Dr. Hastings, she described "the indefinite but ambitious plans" that, immediately on her arrival in Paris, Katherine Olmsted, Chief of the Nursing Division of the League, had outlined for her work "as a four months' advisor on public health". She was to assist in preparing a clear statement of policies for nursing activities of Nursing Bureaus that might also be used by national Red Cross societies and forward it to the national societies in advance of a meeting of the General Council of the League which would begin on 28 April 1924; compile a summary of health nursing programs in various countries, using material in the files of the League, and advise about relationships of the Nursing Bureau with the International Council of Nurses and a European Council of Nursing Education that Mrs. Olmsted had recently helped to create. She was also to study the International Course for Nurses and form an independent judgment of the League's policy with reference to it. Meanwhile she must prepare a series of lectures to be given to the students of the Course. There were other items as well, including the writing of articles for the 'Nursing Supplement' put out by the League, the outlining of talks on practical nursing to be given by graduates of the International Course in their own countries and a course for 'little Mothers' to be used in a similar way. One formidable assignment, to advise about a History of Nursing that would be more acceptable to the Scandinavian and European countries than any currently available, Miss Dyke rejected outright, and she persuaded Mrs. Olmsted to agree to the omission of the history of nursing from the series of lectures that she was to give to the international students. She stipulated also that, without much more knowledge of the countries the students came from, she could not undertake the preparation of material for them to use once they were at home again.

Mrs. Olmsted also explained that, although knowledge of conditions of nursing in France was indispensable to the future plans of the Division, she had not yet had opportunity to study the situation, and appointments had been made for Miss Dyke to do so. During the month of February, therefore, she visited hospitals in various centres throughout the country where nurse-training programs existed and discovered a highly complex pattern. Little wonder Mrs. Olmsted had shied away from it. There were three rival French Red Cross societies which conducted training schools for "benevolent nurses", but in Miss Dyke's words, they had not bridged the barrier between 'benevolent' and 'professional'. Moreover, there were remnants of American influence from nursing activities during World War I that many French nurses resented. For instance, they resented the Florence Nightingale School in Bordeaux where British and American methods predominated, and where American nurses had built a nurses' residence in memory of American and French nurses who died during the World War. In addition, the Ministry of Health had recently issued a decree defining standards of nursing education and had established a "Conseil de Perfectionnement" to enforce them. Although *le conseil* included representatives of the nurses, its existence seemed to many of them to have introduced an element of compulsion. Miss

Dyke also found that French policies and methods, which she thought were a natural development from the origins of nursing in the country, created problems for the League's bureau, because they were not "looked upon with favour" by Scandinavian, English and American nurses.

A further complication from Katherine Olmsted's point of view was the pervasive influence of the Rockefeller Foundation. Elizabeth Crowell, who directed the Foundation's nursing activities in Europe, had been closley identified with nursing in France since 1918 and had recently prepared a report on the subject for the French Ministry of Health. Furthermore, hospitals in nine cities had received aid from the Foundation in the form of resident scholarships, salaries for supervision and teaching, the installation of demonstration rooms and facilities for training in tuberculosis dispensary work. The list was formidable: in 1922, *L'Ecole des Infirmières de l'Assistance Publique de Paris* had been granted eight scholarships of one-year duration for postgraduate work in England; plans were in the making for a public health scholarship at the University of Toronto Department of Nursing for a student from the Bordeaux school, and the Strasbourg school had been promised a fellowship for study of bedside nursing, six months to be spent in England and six months in the United States. Also, both the Lille and Lyon schools had had scholarships for a year's study of hospital organization and administration in England.[4]

Mrs. Olmsted was also embarrassed because Miss Crowell had intimated that she would be willing to assist with the nursing programs of the League, but had made it clear that she did not approve of the International Course as it was being carried on. Moreover, she thought that methods of nursing in Britain, America and Scandinavia were not suitable for Europe, and ignoring the League, she had chosen Toronto instead of London as the place for some types of European nurses to study public health nursing.

When Miss Dyke had completed her "observations and conferences in France", she read the report that Miss Crowell had prepared for the Ministry of Health, and as a result, decided that any report she might make would be inadequate in comparison. "I realize," she wrote, "that interpretation of the situation is so difficult and so important in the development of International and French nursing standards, that I hesitate to submit the immature report which mine would be."

Instead, she recommended that "the three French Red Cross societies unite to appoint an investigator to study and report on the development of nursing in France during the past century". In support of this suggestion, she argued that England and America needed to understand "the original methods of nurse education" that were in process of development in France. In her judgment, the French point of view was needed "to overcome weaknesses of the system in those countries". At the same time, European countries, many of which shared the interest in health and social work that had been "a powerful influence" in France, could benefit from understanding that emphasis and its application to nursing care in hospitals as well as in the hospital training of nurses. Miss Dyke believed that such a survey would help to remove the sense of compulsion many of the nurses had felt as a result of the recent decree of the Ministry of Health. Moreover, she thought that the French Red Cross societies should appoint the investigator. Their interest in developing health nursing would lead to gradual acceptance of the high ethical standards of Red Cross nurses. Lastly, she advocated that *L'infirmière Française*, the French journal of nursing, should include a regular forum on nursing in order to cultivate "a spirit of unity in diversity" between nurses who served gratuitously and those who were employed as professionals by public and philanthropic agencies.[5]

Without any record of Katherine Olmsted's response to these suggestions nor any acknowledgment of Miss Crowell's influence on Miss Dyke's thinking, there remains the nagging question of why she failed to submit a detailed report of her own observations. Surely such evasion of responsibility demeaned her own capacity and was an affront to Mrs. Olmsted, who was already under a cloud of criticism. The latter's appointment had been strongly opposed by "representative American nurses", and some of the officials of the Society who were closely associated with the Nursing Bureau thought she lacked "the mental and administrative qualities" needed for the exacting post she held. This information, given to Miss Dyke in confidence, may have influenced her attitude toward Mrs. Olmsted.

84

About the month she spent in England, where she was doubtless more at home, Miss Dyke wrote a long report,[6] but her experience was marred by strained relationships with Mrs. Carter, who was responsible for the International Course. Also, she found the practice of health nursing as she saw it in London harmfully restricted and without influence in the community. In her view it was lacking in two essentials, the systematic keeping of records and provision for follow-up visits to keep the nurses in touch with patients and make possible health teaching in the homes. She felt the lack of focus and direction that an experienced nurse-supervisor could have provided, and there was little opportunity for exchange of experience among nurses who supervised the field work of students in the International Course. Talking with Mrs. Carter about the matter, she expressed apprehension of these shortcomings as she saw them and, to her dismay, later learned that Mrs. Carter had been discussing her criticisms with the students. To Miss Dyke this seemed a violation of confidence that she feared might "spoil the delightful spirit and confidence of the class". She decided, therefore, to say nothing further about negative impressions and to concentrate on finding out whether the English nurses were aware of the limitations imposed upon their work. Perhaps she would discern ways in which they might be overcome. She had hoped to visit a large number of health agencies, not only for her own interest but also for the benefit of the League, but now her intention had been thwarted — or so she seemed to think.

In her report she described practices that were the basis of her criticisms. For instance, at Guy's Hospital, where students were assigned to a pre-natal clinic, she saw a well-conducted clinic but no evidence of home visiting either before or after attendance at the clinic. Similarly, although the venereal disease clinic at St. Thomas's Hospital was well conducted, the nurses' responsibility ended there. The international students were treated courteously, but no one seemed to realize that in their home countries they would be responsible for organizing programs of public health of which clinical work would be only a part. When Miss Dyke later learned that the role of St. Thomas's nurses was limited to clinic management and treatment, all 'follow-up' being left to the almoner, she realized why the nurses failed to see the task in broader perspective. However, she was less inclined to excuse the almost universal lack of record-keeping.

During visits to two schools she was horrified to find that the nurses' records dealt with nothing but vermin, and teachers whom she talked with thought the nurses' role was simply to rid the pupils' heads of lice. Moreover, even though the school nurse assisted the doctors with the examining of pupils, she had no responsibility to follow through with parents in order to gain their understanding and cooperation, and no case records were kept. In Bethnal Green she was present at a 'necessitous clinic' while the nurse superintendent and her assistant interviewed almost 200 mothers about obtaining free or partially free milk if their income came within 'the graded scale'. The superintendent's rapport with the mothers impressed her as did the team play among the staff, but she saw only one case record with evidence of a home visit.

Nevertheless, she admired the quality of many of the English nurses, one of whom she described as "an ideal public health nurse who would welcome broader interests". She was impressed, too, by evidence of concern to establish high standards among members of the Matrons' Association in the meeting she attended in Leicester. "I am quite sure," she wrote, "that new ideas in nurse education will not be killed by that Association." She noted, too, that she thought the Constitution of the Association would admit Mrs. Carter, implying that such a connection would be helpful for the director of the international course.

A 'Post-Graduate Week' organized by the Public Health Section of the Royal College of Nursing at which she had been invited to speak also won her praise: "Over 170 nurses were enrolled, their expenses paid by their departments with the consent of the Ministry of Health". Miss Dyke was, nevertheless, inhibited on this occasion by constraints, self-imposed or otherwise, under which she worked. Both Miss Rundle, Secretary of the College, and Mrs. Carter had urged her to speak about Toronto. She agreed to do so but felt that she could not speak freely and to avoid the possibility of being misquoted, she wrote her speech and read it to the audience without comment.

Perhaps over-sensitive, she had come to believe that she

was making one gaffe after another. When she encountered a physician associated with the London County Council who agreed that the functions of the health nurses were unnecessarily limited, she asked him whether it might be possible to have directors of public health nursing appointed in London boroughs to supervise the nurses employed by the Council. Mrs. Carter cautioned her, however, that such a question might be unwise, since she knew nothing about the doctor's relationship to the London County Council staff. At the same time, Mrs. Carter was urging her to stress the importance of giving the nurses more responsibility. In further conversations with physicians, therefore, she merely mentioned that "nothing corresponding to a matron in a hospital existed in the health field".

Although Miss Dyke became increasingly reluctant "to say anything a foreigner should not say", if she felt some empathy with an individual, she seems to have been more forthright and on occasion "took advantage of opportunities to use Dr. Hastings' policies to illustrate points of discussion". She confined herself, however, to consideration of nursing service, and even when the Bradford Medical Director of Health asked her to describe the plan of organization she would like to see, she thought it unwise "to go beyond expressing the wish for a director for public health nursing". Yet she was ambivalent about this inhibition for she considered the work in Bradford the best she had seen and would have liked to have said so. At the same time she wished she might have added that she could never endorse a policy of administration that identified the health visitor with poverty or 'border line' cases. Like Dr. Hastings, she believed that public health was a concern of the entire community and that the services of a public health nurse should not be restricted to so-called 'charity cases'.

When Miss Dyke returned to Paris, Mrs. Olmsted told her that Mrs. Carter had been seriously depressed by her visit, but although duly penitent, Miss Dyke wrote a lengthy explanation of what she had tried to accomplish and the difficulties she had had. She felt that her stay in London had not been easy for either herself or Mrs. Carter. The visit should not have been scheduled at examination time and then, her relations with Mrs. Carter had been strained by what she felt to have been a betrayal of confidence. She was also critical of Mrs. Carter for selecting institutions for field work without having first visited them. Furthermore, that Mrs. Carter neither conferred with field supervisors nor required reports from them seemed to her reprehensible. Nevertheless, she expressed admiration for Mrs. Carter's personal relations with the students. She was "a student with students ... mother of the group and Director of the Course". Moreover, she was "painfully aware of her own inexperience" — a not improbable result of Miss Dyke's thinly disguised disapproval.

The two women had also been at odds about the role of the Director of the International Course and the place of the Course in the curriculum of Bedford College. Lectures were being given by the College Department of Social Science, but no attempt had been made to create new lectures or even to modify old ones to meet the needs and interests of international students. Mrs. Carter had supplemented the lectures by enlisting speakers on particular subjects, but, although Miss Dyke herself had been one of these, such a plan seemed to her of doubtful value. She saw the task of the League of Red Cross Societies as one of assisting students to take advantage of learning opportunities in London or elsewhere according to individual needs. This type of program would require a department of nursing directed by a nurse but should not, in her opinion, be a department of Bedford College. Part of the problem, she felt, was that Mrs. Carter had failed to see that the role of the director of nurse education in the International Course was not the same as that "generally accepted by those responsible for educational courses". However, she, with others who were aware of the situation, had tried without success to help Mrs. Carter recognize the nature of the task of educating student nurses from diverse backgrounds and with differing levels of education and experience.

Miss Dyke's recommendations covered a broad scope, the chief one being that the League should establish an international centre for nurse education in London with a residence and a nurse director. The director of the centre should confer with schools and colleges that offered hospital and postgraduate courses "with a view to modifying the regular lectures and the practical experience as the needs of each student and her community indicate". The success of such a centre, she believed, would require continuing cooperation with Bedford College, King's College, and the Royal College of Nursing. Further, she suggested an approach to either the British Red Cross Society or to the Rockefeller Foundation for assistance in developing a model plan of public health nursing in a London borough or even a department of nursing in Bedford College.

Meanwhile, she liked the plan that was afoot for the ensuing year to offer two international courses, one in public health nursing and the other in hospital administration, with students of both courses living in the same residence. She thought this plan would provide a sound basis for developing an international centre of broader scope.

Not surprisingly, Mrs. Carter was less than enthusiastic about these recommendations, but the crunch came when Mrs. Olmsted declared that they would destroy the International Course. She accused Miss Dyke of working with Elizabeth Crowell "to send nurses to Toronto who should go to London". In anger, Miss Dyke retorted that what Mrs. Olmsted wanted was a rubber stamp, not an advisor, and she withdrew her carefully compiled report from the files, fearing that Mrs. Olmsted's attitude toward the recommendations might "lead her to use the report unwisely".

To Dr. Hastings, Miss Dyke wrote a full account of her experience in both France and England, not omitting the altercation with Katherine Olmsted. She explained, however, that the arrival of Miss Fox, the nurse who represented the American Red Cross on Mrs. Olmsted's committee, had saved the day and opened the way for her to attend the meeting of the committee in an advisory capacity. She reported, also, that in the end, the recommendations that were sent to the General Council were in line with her thinking. Moreover, Mrs. Olmsted had come round to thinking that the International Course, 'her baby', had been rescued.

To the Baroness Mannerheim, Chairman of the Nursing Advisory Board of the League, Miss Dyke sent a detailed review of her experience in London, including her reservations about the existing arrangements for the International Course. She enclosed both the recommendations of the advisory committee and a copy of her letter to Dr. Hastings explaining that she had written to him because she felt it necessary to keep her home people fully informed in case she might need to send them an 'S.O.S.' Was she really thinking she might need to call for help, or did she perchance ponder the possibility of being invited to join the staff of the League? In the handwritten postscript to her letter to Dr. Hastings (omitted from her letter to the Baroness), she intimated that she thought she might be asked to act in a temporary capacity during reorganization, but assured Dr. Hastings that she did not wish to do so.

In that same letter to Dr. Hastings there is a hint of explanation of the constraints she had worked under and her wariness about possible misuse of her recommendations: " ... it is necessary for me to remember that my appointment was not approved by the Canadian Red Cross". She seems not to have been informed that on 1 February 1924, at its earliest meeting after her appointment, the Executive Committee of the Canadian Red Cross Society had passed a motion that a message be sent to the League "expressing the opinion that Miss Dyke is well qualified to give advice on public health nursing".[7] She probably did know, however, that two days had gone by after the newspaper announcement of her appointment before the Canadian Red Cross Society received a cable from Sir Claude Hill, Director General of the League, announcing the appointment. That circumstance was in itself embarrassing, but, if, by chance, she had seen the 'tongue in cheek' reply of the General Secretary, she might have been even less sure of the backing of the Canadian Society. He referred to the delay in arrival of the cable and added: "So far as information and experience are concerned you certainly could not have invited anyone more calculated to assist you and from this standpoint I do not see how anyone could object to your choice".

By now, three months had gone by since she had arrived in Paris, long enough for her to have lost touch with colleagues and friends at home. The only letter from Toronto among her papers is one from Kathleen Russell, in which there is reference to an earlier one from Nora Moore about a meeting of hospital superintendents when arrangements between the Department of Health and the nurse-training schools had been discussed "in a frosty atmosphere".[8] Eventually, however, discussion had turned to the main topic, whether pupil-nurse work could be arranged through the

University Department of Public Health Nursing. There were practical difficulties to be overcome, but Miss Russell had offered to make every effort to enrol a group in the autumn, though Miss Gunn had cautioned against any new arrangement unless there was "some reasonable hope of permanence". Miss Russell also mentioned the problems of combining theoretical and practical work. She had concluded that, without minimizing the importance of practical field work, there must be greater emphasis on the theory of nursing. She realized that the subject could not be discussed satisfactorily in a letter, but she wanted to keep Miss Dyke informed because she was currently so closely involved with the League of Red Cross Societies in planning for the training of nurses.

The letter reflects a cordial relationship between the two women who, while they shared a concern for high quality of education for nurses, did not agree about the relative importance of theoretical background and nursing practice in curriculum.[9] Miss Russell may have anticipated that Miss Dyke might oppose changes that seemed to her undue limitations on field work experience. In any case, the letter was a thin thread of communication, and there is no evidence of a reply from Miss Dyke. Writing to Dr. Hastings, she raised the question of having an additional month's leave and asked for a reply by cable. Whether Dr. Hastings agreed to such an extension is uncertain, but the letter ended on a note of nostalgia. She wrote, "I am very homesick for the Department ..., and am eager to share again in the development of the work in Toronto". The letter ended,

Respectfully yours,
Eunice Dyke.
The international interlude had come to an end.

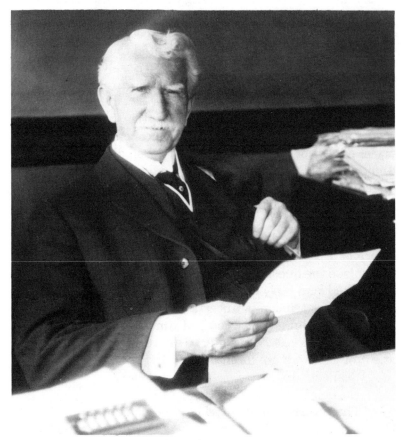

Dr. C.J.O. Hastings, Medical Officer of Health in 1925

Chapter Five

After Paris

Returning to Share in Further Developments

Happy, no doubt, to have returned, Miss Dyke found much to be done to broaden and deepen the services of the Division of Public Health Nursing, and her eight remaining years as Director of the Division saw important new developments as well as the continuance of former responsibilities and sporadic epidemics to be coped with. Her conviction that the family was the essential unit in health work continued to be a guiding principle, with emphasis on the health care of children at every stage of life.

The baby clinics, later called child health centres, still provided guidance and care for the health of growing numbers of infants and pre-schoolers. Attendance increased year by year until 1932 the numbers were beyond the capacity of the nurses to meet demands, and an appointment system was introduced resulting in decreased attendance but much improved service.[1] Literature for general distribution continued to be one of the chief educational instruments of the Division. A pamphlet entitled *Pre-Natal care – Advice to the Expectant Mother*, published in 1922, had stressed the principle that every child had the right to a healthy birth. Later this material was expanded in two publications in red covers that were called 'The Red Books'. By 1931, one of these, *The Care of the Infant and Young Child*, had been reprinted 17 times. It gave a mother guidance in such details of care as feeding, bathing, clothing and habit training as well as information about children's diseases. Both pamphlets were prepared under the direction of the Division's Supervisor of Child Welfare and approved by the Medical Director of The

93

Hospital for Sick Children. *The Expectant Mother*, which had been approved by a professor of Obstetrics and Gynaecology in the University of Toronto, was published separately in 1927. It described the evidences of pregnancy, explained possible complications, and how to sustain mental and physical health, and directed attention to the responsibilities of both parents. In harmony with Miss Dyke's conviction, it indicated a special appeal to the mother:

> You must remember that your baby is dependent upon you for its physical and mental development. This life is entrusted to your care; if you guard it with devotion and intelligence, you have accomplished the greatest duty allotted to womankind.[2]

In this 'post-Paris' period, a coordinated community service for families stricken with illness came to fruition after several years of planning. It was a scheme for visiting housekeepers that the nurses under Miss Dyke's leadership had dreamed of as at least a partial solution of the crisis a family faced if the mother were ill and the children without supervision. Often the services of a trained nurse were needed for only part of a day, but there was need of a person who, following the nurse's instructions, could carry on the care of the patient and help the family weather the emergency. Social workers shared the nurses' concern. In their opinion, there were also families with a mother who was not a good manager but able to learn, if a capable person were available to work with her for a short time.

The problem was first tackled in an organized way in October 1921 when the Federation for Community Service convened a meeting of representatives of health and welfare agencies to explore ways of dealing with it. Eunice Dyke was there and also Jean Gunn of the Toronto General Hospital and Kathleen Russell, by then head of the University Department of Nursing, as well as equally well known social workers and several interested volunteers. The consensus of the group was that there should be a corps of specially trained domestic workers, mature women who had coped with similar situations in their own families.

Committee work continued well into 1922 and, although extensive enquiry yielded the information that "no similar service was discoverable in other communities", the group was not deterred. By July, having worked out an estimate of costs and a plan for training the workers, in which Miss Dyke was involved, they proposed a one-year experiment under the sponsorship of either the Department of Public Health or the Federation for Community Service. Nothing more happened, however, until April 1924, when a meeting of representatives of the interested agencies was called at the request of Dr. George Smith, President of the Toronto Branch of the Canadian Red Cross Society, who announced that a sum of money and a house previously given to the Toronto Nursing Mission had been offered to the Red Cross for some welfare purpose. The Society had decided to accept the gift and use it for the kind of service that had been recommended earlier. This time, Miss Dyke still being abroad, Dr. Hastings attended the meeting and spoke for the Department of Public Health.

There was general rejoicing at the windfall, but there remained one obstacle to be overcome. The late Goldwin Smith, who had owned the house, had willed the residue of his estate to Cornell University, and questions relating to transfer of the property were still to be solved. By March 1925, however, deeds of the house had been received and registered, and a committee under the chairmanship of Barbara Blackstock (later Mrs. H.J. Cody) undertook to oversee the planning, including the search for a director who, it was agreed, should be a household science graduate trained in nutrition and household management. Lexa Denne, a University of Toronto household science graduate, who had had teaching experience in technical schools in Vancouver and Toronto and in the Evangelia Settlement House, was appointed to the post. A small group took over the furnishing and equipping of the house as a headquarters and a home centre for workers who could arrange to live there. By May 1925, five women were enrolled in the first training class. Miss Denne taught household management, budgeting, nutrition and special diets, and a public health nurse was brought in to give instruction in home nursing and child care. Everything well in hand, the official opening was held on 16 June. The workers were to be called Visiting Housekeepers, and the responsible committee was known as the Visiting Housekeepers Committee of the Toronto Branch of the Canadian Red Cross Society.

Miss Dyke kept in close touch with these developments, in particular the training course which, at least on one occasion, she arranged to have extended to include an 'outsider'. Janet Holmes, who spent many years as a missionary in Bolivia, tells of Miss Dyke persuading her to take the course as part of her preparation for work in the mission field. She remembers that most of the students were mature women, although a few were younger. They 'lived in', and she felt herself at some disadvantage to have to go from her family home for early classes. However, the experience proved invaluable. She learned skills that proved useful not only in caring for her own household but also, in her work with Bolivian women, and now, more than half a century later, she is still grateful for Miss Dyke's foresight, which also encompassed a visit to the Women's College Hospital to see the birth of a baby. Once in a remote place in Bolivia, where there was neither a doctor nor a midwife available, Miss Holmes was the only one to help a mother in the delivery of her baby.

The Visiting Housekeepers' service soon justified its existence, and financial responsibility for its continuance was transferred to the Federation for Community Service, with a continuing grant from the Red Cross for work with families of ex-service men and help from the city for families on relief. When the transfer was completed in 1929, the agency was re-named the Housekeepers' Association of Toronto, and Barbara Blackstock was elected President. Meanwhile similar services were being organized under Red Cross auspices all across Canada, and visiting homemakers (the name was changed in 1934), whether paid out of public funds or by individual clients, were increasingly recognized as women who provide an indispensable service in the community.[3] Miss Dyke maintained an interest in the Association and in her later years sought to have its scope extended to provide assistance for the elderly to enable them to remain in their own homes.

Control of communicable diseases continued to be an urgent and recurring problem. Since 1919, in addition to the medical program in schools and baby clinics, individuals and families going to subsidized summer camps had been inspected by a district medical health officer with the assistance of a district nurse. Despite such precautions, however, sporadic epidemics occurred, often among children. In 1926, to cope systematically with the problem in all its aspects, Elsie Hickey, one of Miss Dyke's ablest nurses, was made special supervisor of acute communicable disease nursing. April of that year brought epidemics of whooping cough, measles and diphtheria and in the early fall an outbreak of poliomyelitis among children of one to five years. Ever since 1890 'polio' had been known to be contagious, and, therefore a public health problem. From 1910 to 1913, it had occurred in every state of the United States and every province of Canada, affecting adults as well as children, often leaving crippled limbs and faces in a perpetual grimace. It continued to be a chronic scourge until 1955, when testing proved Dr. J.E. Salk's vaccine to be an immunizing agent for from 80 to 90 percent of known cases. In 1926, only isolation of its victims could check an epidemic, and the Department of Public Health took immediate action to that end, with the public health nurses in the forefront. Despite their best efforts, however, there were 13 'polio' deaths out of 38 registered cases, and 37 deaths resulted from whooping cough.[4] Among those who survived the former disease were many who were disabled for life. Diphtheria took 89 lives, but new hope was found in the use of toxoid, given for the first time in a large public school when the principal and the public health nurse were alarmed by the prevalence of the disease in the school district. The success of the experiment led to the organizing of toxoid teams in all city schools in 1929.[5] Measles, too, was by then under better control; out of a total of 2,344 cases in 1926, there were only 12 fatalities.

Most demanding of Miss Hickey's responsibilities was the supervision of the care of venereal disease patients. An Act for the Prevention of Venereal Disease passed by the Ontario Legislature in 1918 had laid the basis for a comprehensive program for treatment of venereal diseases, including special clinics in hospitals and the service of public health nurses. In Toronto, clinics had been opened in six large hospitals, and public health nurses from the Hospital Social Service unit of the Department of Public Health were appointed to the clinics to encourage regular attendance of patients and inquire into sources and contacts. Selected cases were referred to district nursing staff or to suitable social agencies, and plans for clinical treatment were reported to agencies that had referred patients for diagnosis and treatment. The amount of help that could be asked of private agencies was limited, however, because of the need for privacy in order to maintain the confidence of the public and safeguard the trust of private physicians who referred patients to the clinic. It was a service that required sensitive insight on the part of the supervising nurse and the staff under her direction.[6]

For now almost two decades, in all their varied activities, the public health nurses had worked closely with the N.W.A. secretaries, one of whom was still placed in each district office. "The nurses profited by daily contact with trained social workers, and they found advantage in the nurses' viewpoint", wrote Zada Keefer. In 1927 the value of this cooperation was underlined when two social workers and a volunteer from the American Association for Organizing Family Social Work (later known as The Family Service Association of America) made a survey of family social work in Toronto, under the auspices of the Federation for Community Service. Their study had convinced the visitors of "the fine partnership" between nurses and social workers which they attributed to "the generous arrangement of sharing offices with the public health nurses as hostesses". They noted that the average family in illness turned instinctively to the physician and the nurse and welcomed "instruction along preventive lines" but they hesitated to call upon the help of the social worker in a problem of child training, economic need, or estrangement between members of the family. That being the case in general, they had found that Toronto's public health nurses were able to recognize "evidences of family disruption and subtle symptoms of trouble ahead" that indicated need for the services of the social worker. On the other hand, however, "there was not quite so much evidence . . . that the social worker understood the field of public health". To correct this lack, the report suggested that "a course of instruction in the fundamental principles of health and recognition of significant health conditions should be open to social workers", the purpose being "to sharpen their perception of the symptoms of ill-health".[7] Miss Dyke, who so strongly believed in cooperation between the two professions and who was convinced that the family was the essential unit in the health and welfare of the community, was deeply gratified by this report, and she was confident in a sense of the rightness of the focus of her work.

Over the years Miss Dyke had kept in touch with voluntary organizations, in order to acquaint a wider public with the role of the public health nurses and stimulate action to improve the health of the community. One such relationship that she valued highly was with the Local Council of Women. Not only had she joined it as an individual member, but she had also encouraged the public health nurses' council to become an affiliate organization. In 1928, however, Dr. Hastings requested that the nurses' council withdraw from affiliation with both the Local Council of Women and the Home and School Association. His explanation for this decision was that misquotation of the nurses, who were employees of the City, might lead to undue criticism of the Department of Public Health.[8]

Even without firm evidence to support the assumption, one is led to think there may have been some connection between this decision of Dr. Hastings and an assignment entrusted to Miss Dyke by the Canadian Nurses' Association two years earlier. In November 1926, representing the CNA at an executive conference of the National Council of Women, she had been a member of a committee to study maternity bonuses. As a result of this experience, she perceived similarity between the Council's problems in relating to its provincial and local counterparts and those of the CNA in dealing with its parallel affiliates. She saw hazards for both national bodies in that the influence of their local units tended to be weakened "by an attempt to unify from national offices down rather than from 'the home town up'". In the matter of maternity bonuses, for instance, conflict had arisen as a result of a new policy of using expert consultants instead of the former practice of acting on suggestions from provincial and local councils, often without adequate research having been done by qualified committees.

At the November meeting of the National Council of Women, a resolution in favour of maternity bonuses had been referred to a special committee on which the Canadian Medical Association, the Canadian Nurses Association and the recently organized Canadian Association of Social Workers[9] were to be represented. Before this committee had met to deal with the matter, however, a plan for maternity bonuses to be submitted to provincial and national governments had been approved by the sub-executive and forwarded to local councils. "It is evident that the present situation within the National Council of Women leads to premature action in matters calling for the most expert advice Canada has to offer," wrote Miss Dyke. At the same time, she commended the Toronto Local Council of Women for having appointed a social service advisory committee that was prepared to study any social project under consideration. Professional workers were thus given opportunity to influence legislation and public service. Here, Miss Dyke thought, was a challenge for the nursing profession, and she wrote:

> The nurses' relationship to the community gives a peculiar responsibility for the advancement of social welfare. Are we so organized locally and nationally that we can undertake research work if called upon in the public interest to give advice leading to legislative action?[10]

Was Dr. Hastings alarmed at the prospect of members of his Department becoming involved in such a program, and/or was he apprehensive of Miss Dyke's pursuit of an idea that she was bent upon promoting? The incident occurred at about the same time as a decision taken by Dr. Hastings to disallow educational privileges for nurses to improve their qualifications, a decision which Miss Dyke attributed to his advancing years and failing health.

Another change occurred in 1928, when a division of mental health was formed in the Department of Public Health with Eric Clarke as Director, a position that gave him more scope than he had as consulting psychiatrist. Emma de V. Clarke was transferred from the Division of Public Health Nursing to the new Division but she continued to supervise the mental health work of the nurses. The new Division worked in close cooperation, not only with the Nursing Division but also with the medical service of the Division (later Department) of Social Welfare and the Juvenile Court.[11]

In 1929, Dr. Hastings resigned because of ill health and was succeeded by Dr. Gordon Jackson who had been a medical officer under the Board of Education and who, after the transfer of medical services in the schools, was appointed Medical Officer of Health for the Parkdale District. Whether or not by design, in his monthly reports to the Board of Health, Dr. Jackson gave less attention to public health nursing than Dr. Hastings had done. In addition to the inevitable strain of working under a new chief, the years 1930 and '31 were traumatic for Miss Dyke. Her elder sister, Ethel, Mrs. Jospeh West, died of cancer in August 1930, and while she was gravely ill, Eunice herself contracted the disease. She was 'off service' at intervals during January and March, and in April had an operation for cancer of the colon. Recovery was slow, and she was absent until the end of August. In the following year, her father, 85, died in May, and only a month later her brother Gordon, the youngest of the family and a general favourite, also died, leaving her with a deep sense of loss.

Nevertheless, during those years there were developments in the work of the Nursing Division that were gratifying to her. One of these was in the field of maternal care which had long been a special concern. As early as 1918, a professor of obstetrics in the University of Toronto had agreed to act as honorary director of maternal care in the Department of Public Health. This innovation, which provided ready access to expert medical advice, was possible because of Dr. Hastings' close relationship with the University. Despite continuing efforts to cope with the problem, however, by 1930, the incidence of maternal mortality had reached alarming proportions, and a conference of nurses from the Department of Public Health, the Victorian Order and the St. Elizabeth Association of Visiting Nurses was held to try to achieve more effective cooperation in maternal services. This event was closely related to other noteworthy undertakings with similar purpose. During the winter of 1930-31, a joint committee of the Local Council of Women and the Child Welfare Council of Toronto organized a campaign to awaken the public to the needs and problems of mothers. In March the Board of Health took up the matter and asked the Medical Officer of Health to bring in a report on maternal mortality, including recommendations for action. Mothers' Day that year was devoted to the broader question of maternal welfare, and a mass meeting under the auspices of the Local Council of Women and the Child Wel-

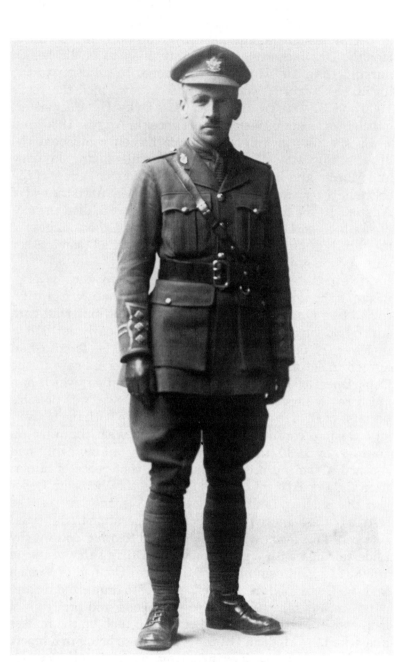

Capt. Frederick Gordon Dyke, W.W. I

fare Council directed the attention of citizens to the subject.[12]

The Medical Officer of Health presented his report on 31 August, and the Chairman of the Board of Health called a conference of all interested organizations to plan a strategy for dealing with the matter. At the Conference, held on 30 September 1931, there were representatives from the Academy of Medicine, the Victorian Order, the St. Elizabeth Association, the Visiting Housekeepers' Association, the Mothercraft Society, the Local Council of Women, the Child Welfare Council and the Department of Public Health, including Dr. Jackson, his deputy, Dr. L.A. Pequegnat, and several nurses from the Nursing Division.[13] Speeches were limited to 10 minutes, to allow everybody to participate, and it was evident that all the organizations were ready to cooperate to the fullest extent in a campaign to reduce, even eliminate, infant and maternal mortality. There was challenge in the statement that 48 percent of maternal mortality was preventable; in 80 percent of the deaths, the mother had not had any prenatal care. Interestingly enough, it was suggested that the public health bulletin be revived, it having been one of the most effective educational instruments in combatting health hazards. The meeting unanimously agreed to the appointment of an advisory committee comprised of representatives of the concerned organizations to work with the Board of Health. The Chairman named a nominating committee of which Miss Dyke was a member, and later in the month, after intensive study, the Board of Control and the City Council, drawing upon the suggestion of the nominating committee, appointed an advisory committee and three sub-committees to deal respectively with pre-natal, intra-natal and post-natal care. Public health nurses were active in the work of all of these groups and, in the words of Janet Neilson, "learned as much as their mental attitudes permitted about community roles and relationships".

With the onset of economic depression in 1930, the welfare of the growing numbers of unemployed men and women became a major civic concern, and in 1931, a department of public welfare was formed to replace the division that had existed since 1920 in the Department of Public Health. A director, the Commissioner of Public Welfare, and a considerable staff, including a division of family welfare with a supervisor and three family workers, were appointed.[14] The public health nurses were assigned new duties in connection with special diets that were provided by the new Department for individuals who suffered from diabetes, anaemia, malnutrition or other abnormalities affecting their health. Requests for these special diets, prescribed by either private physicians or those in hospital clinics, were sent to district offices of the Nursing Division to be processed. The nurses completed the necessary forms before forwarding them to the Welfare Department and were responsible for supervision of the patients who received the diets. This system, cumbrous though it was, made it possible to meet more adequately the nutritional needs of babies and of pregnant and nursing mothers.

Also, in 1930, arrangements were made for student dietitians who had completed their course of study and were doing part-time practical work in hospitals to spend a month in the Nursing Division. At first only two students were assigned, one to the eastern district and one to the west, but the service proved so helpful, especially for diabetic patients, that it was extended to other districts.

By 1931, the Division of Public Health Nursing had a staff of 115 nurses, a corps of civil servants to be taken into account in the City of Toronto. Able, well-trained women working from nine district offices, they were aware of medical and social needs in the areas of the city for which they were responsible and were frequently consulted by both members of other divisions of the Department of Public Health and representatives of city-wide agencies concerned with the health and welfare of the community. Eunice Dyke's days in the Department were, however, approaching an end that she had not anticipated. By dint of unrelenting effort and her vision of building an effective instrument of public health nursing in Toronto, she had made a notable contribution to the community. It may have been a merciful fate that spared her the trauma of seeing the staff reduced by 12 nurses in 1933, when economic depression led to rigorous cut-backs in the City's budget.

Chapter Six

The Consuming Concern

Education for Public Health Nursing

Public health nurses must be carefully selected and thoroughly trained if they are to succeed.   *Eunice H. Dyke*

Special education for public health nurses had been a consuming concern for Miss Dyke throughout the years she spent in the Toronto Department of Public Health. She knew that preparation for a distinctive role in the promotion of health and the prevention of disease in the community was essential for public health nursing and, since her first responsibility was to and for the nurses of her own Division, there she must begin. So it was that her inventive mind turned to patterns of in-service education. But the problem had wider dimensions. Even before Miss Dyke took up her post in Toronto, vigorous discussion of the education of nurses was well under way in nurses' organizations, local, provincial, and national. Miss Dyke entered into educational planning at all three levels, always pursuing her particular interest in the preparation of public health nurses.

Noon-day discussion lunches in district offices were, in the opinion of Miss Dyke's successors, much the most effective form of in-service education that she began. Except in cases of emergency, all nurses of a district were expected to be present and, because they had been selected from varying backgrounds and were dealing with varying situations, the lunches were an opportunity for fruitful exchange of experience in dealing with day-to-day problems. Visitors invited in rotation from community organizations gave the

105

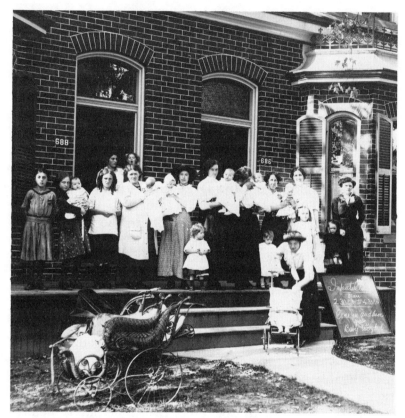

A popular baby weighing clinic in Toronto

discussion still broader scope. They came from related groups with which the nurses were in frequent touch. Most closely involved of these were the social workers of the N.W.A. and other neighbours and colleagues of the nurses. Others came from the Children's Aid Society; the Big Sisters and Big Brothers associations; the Heather and Samaritan clubs; the Victorian Order of Nurses and the St. Elizabeth Nursing Association. Also, teachers and principals from neighbouring schools were often present and district medical health officers joined the lunches in their areas from time to time. Miss Dyke believed that this wider range of participation would foster team play without which individual efforts of the public health nurses would make slight impression on the health of the community. Dr. Hastings became convinced that the lunches were "largely responsible for district *esprit de corps*". They remained an essential feature of the administration for many years after Miss Dyke had left the Division of Public Health Nursing.[1]

The noon-day lunches were begun early in 1914, shortly after the creation of the Division of Public Health Nurses, but already a year earlier, Miss Dyke had initiated another educational instrument, an organization of the nurses called the Public Health Nurses Association. The objective of the Association, described by Florence Emory who was chosen as its president in 1916, was "to further the service in which the nurses were engaged and stimulate their personal growth". At the first meeting held 13 October 1913, there were 17 nurses present, and Miss Dyke was elected president. It was agreed that there be weekly meetings with talks by specialists on some aspect of health or social work and always also 'a question box'. Miss Dyke would either answer the questions or refer them to an outside authority and no question was to be left unanswered. Officers were elected annually, and educational programs of the Association had the approval of the Medical Officer of Health. It was a congenial arrangement, with the nurses feeling free to raise questions and, on occasion, ask Miss Dyke to let them know Dr. Hastings' opinion on an issue.[2] The Association continued until 1919, when it was disbanded to be replaced by the Nurses' Advisory Council comprised of a member from the central office, one from hospital extension (or social) service and one from each district office. The members were to be elected by ballot, and it was recommended that they *not* be district superintendents. The Council met at least three times annually, oftener if necessary, to deal with educational and social matters, including representation at conventions, which had tended to be a perquisite of senior staff.[3]

Also in the autumn of 1913 when Arthur Burnett was appointed to a post in the Division of Public Health Nursing, it was understood that he would assist with the nurses' education in social service for which their hospital training had given them no background. Later, as head of the Division of Social Service, he was given wider scope to develop the social work of the Department of Public Health in relation to other civic and voluntary agencies. Working with the nurses assigned to his Division, Burnett found that the families whom the nurses visited increasingly depended upon them for information about laws and social organizations that affected their lives. In the winter of 1916-17, therefore, he responded to a request from senior nurses of the Department for a series of lectures dealing with such subjects as The Children's Protection Act, the Children's Aid Society, Ontario's Factory acts, duties of the Workmen's Compensation Board and the work of the Trades and Labour Branch of the Ontario Government. He himself gave 15 of the lectures and for the other four, he brought in individuals from outside the Department. It was a measure of the nurses' interest, he believed, that they were present at 8.30 on Tuesday mornings for the entire series.[4]

Further opportunity for formal education was opened to the city's nurses in September 1914, when, following a proposal of President Robert Falconer, the University of Toronto established a department of social service. Falconer's plan was to offer a curriculum adapted to the needs of social service workers that would deal with questions of poverty and philanthropy, crime and prevention, government and administration. Instruction would be given in lectures, discussion sessions and supervised field work.[5] Because most of these subjects related to social problems that the public health nurses encountered in their work, at Dr. Hastings' request, they were admitted to two courses: The Field of Social Work, and Medical Social Service. Classes met on Mondays and Thursdays at 4.30 throughout the academic year, and each course included about 25 hours of instruction. The nurses took the examinations set by the University, and credit was given for satisfactory completion of the work, a record being kept of individual standings. It was an arrangement that was particularly gratifying to Miss Dyke, the first step toward professional training for her nurses. With minor changes the plan was continued until, in 1920, the University introduced a certificate course in public health nursing, forerunner of the present Faculty of Nursing.

The prospectus of the new University Department of Social Service listed two courses to be given by A.H. Burnett, the content of which suggests the scope of his interests. He was to lecture on The Family and the Community and lead a discussion course on Charities. Miss Dyke felt that his association with the University soon claimed Burnett's first allegiance. Believing that his chief interest was to promote himself personally, she resented his behaviour. "He calls himself the man of the hour," she wrote. Years later, recalling the past, she charged that he had lacked interest in developing the capacities of the nurses. She admitted, however, that his work at the University was remembered gratefully by some of his early students, but added, "It is doubtful whether he worked for the strengthening of that organization apart from himself". In her eyes, his resignation in 1917 had been "a relief to the Department".[6]

In the fall of 1915, Miss Dyke herself began nine months' study leave in Boston. She enrolled in a course in Public Health Nursing scheduled from 22 September 1915 to 6 June 1916 that was offered by Simmons College in affiliation with the Instructive District Nursing Association (incorporated in 1882 to provide nurses who, as well as caring for the sick, would teach their families or friends the elements of hygiene and home nursing) and the School for Social Workers. The Instructive District Nursing Association had begun a short course in public health nursing for student and graduate nurses from selected hospitals in 1906 and later, in response to demand for more thorough preparation, arranged for the more comprehensive course in cooperation with Simmons College and the School for Social Workers. Simmons College taught the theoretical background, "the fundamental principles upon which the public

health sciences, including preventive medicine, are based",
and the School for Social Workers offered lectures and conferences on principles of social service and the history of public
health nursing. The latter included developments in tuberculosis and infant welfare nursing, industrial nursing,
school nursing and mental hygiene, with emphasis on organization and administration. Students spent seven hours a
week in field work with a social work agency and visits to
selected institutions, then wrote reports and attended conferences as 'follow-up'. The Instructive District Nursing
Association, which stressed preventive medicine, arranged
for students to have experience in working with patients for
whom general well-being rather than illness was the focus of
concern, and if possible, each student worked with the same
family during the entire period of the course. There were
also opportunities to observe school nursing and the care of
tuberculosis patients. The tuition fee was $80.00, and Sim-
mons College granted certificates to those who completed
the work satisfactorily.[7]

An anonymous journal of the period, now in the
archives of Simmons College, lists Eunice Dyke of Toronto
among students of the course, but she left no record of the
experience, valuable as it must have been. At a later period
of her life, however, Mary Beard, a well known public health
nurse who at the time was Director of the Instructive District Nursing Association, proved to be her trusted friend
and adviser.

Meanwhile, in Toronto, as had already been agreed
before Miss Dyke left for Boston, a two-week preliminary
period of field work was made compulsory for candidates
seeking appointment to the public health nursing staff, in
order to orient them to community work. Supervision of this
additional training, which began in October, was at first
assigned to the superintendent of Moss Park District, but
soon to ease the load, some of the candidates were sent to
each district, and responsibility for supervision was shared
among all the superintendents. Later, during the first year
she was on staff, each nurse was required to take the medical social work course offered by the University and pass the
examination set by the University. If a nurse were appointed
in mid-year, Miss Dyke or whoever temporarily replaced her
as Director of the Division helped the newcomer to make

special arrangements with the University for admission to classes.

Dr. Hastings frequently gathered the nurses together on Saturday mornings, when regular work was less pressing, and spoke to them about their role, as members of the only division of the Department of Public Health that provided personal services in a program of preventive medicine. Moreover, in these talks, he never failed to stress women's suitability for the task to which the public health nurses were committed. Then, early in 1916, all employees of the Department participated in a course that he had planned "to embrace every branch of the work of the Department and the outside branches with which it cooperated closely". This latter experience gave the nurses knowledge of the scope of public health work in the city and assured them that their share in it was understood by their colleagues in other branches of city government. From time to time also, they had the advantage of medical lectures by specialists in various fields; tuberculosis, child hygiene and welfare, minor skin diseases and the handling of clinics. As well, occasional demonstrations arranged in cooperation with hospital staff gave them practical assistance in such matters as infant feeding and the care of orthopaedic patients. In 1917, the district superintendents were admitted to lectures given on Saturday mornings for clinic physicians at the Hospital for Sick Children.

It would appear that these educative experiences were seldom evaluated objectively. But at the end of a series of lectures on tuberculosis given by Dr. J.H. Elliott in February 1917, Miss Dyke asked the nurses for individual written statements of their opinion of the lectures, which Dr. Elliott thought should have been known to them before they assumed the duties of tuberculosis nursing. However, there is no record of either the replies of the nurses or whether Dr. Elliott's suggestion for such preliminary preparation was accepted.

In the fall of 1917, it was agreed with Dr. Franklin Johnson of the University Department of Social Service that the city nurses should no longer take his introductory course on social work, a decision, Miss Dyke reported, that Dr. Johnson had welcomed. He had planned it as a university course for full-time students of social work but now felt that it had not been satisfactory for the nurses, an opinion Miss Dyke, herself, had come to share. In the previous term, at the request of the nurses she had asked Dr. Johnson to exempt them from writing an essay on 'The Wayward Girl'. They complained that Dr. Johnson was morbid in his tendency to concentrate on social problems arising from sexual relationships, but they seem not to have noted that the girl was considered the culprit. In reporting this matter to Dr. Hastings, Miss Dyke mentioned that Miss Hall of the Victorian Order had had similar criticism of Dr. Johnson from her nurses. However, the matter was not mentioned as a factor in the decision to discontinue the course.

As a result of the work of Robert M. MacIver, who succeeded Dr. Johnson in 1918, Miss Dyke's estimate of the direction of the Department of Social Service rose substantially. Dr. MacIver was a Scot from Aberdeen University, who had joined the faculty of the University in 1915 as associate professor of political economy. In June 1919 a letter to President Falconer expressing appreciation of his service as Director of the Department of Social Service included signatures of the Department of Public Health nurses, including Miss Dyke. A resolution from 'Social Service Alumni' under the same date, signed by Kathleen Russell among others, praised his achievement in linking the Department of Social Service more closely with the University, the community and the social forces of Canada and the United States. It also voiced the hope that he might continue as Director of the Department.[8]

As a student at The Johns Hopkins School for Nurses, Miss Dyke had learned the importance of keeping up-to-date with developments in the nursing profession. Now, aware of the ever-increasing body of literature in the field, she saw that books and articles relating to their work were brought to the attention of the nurses. Gradually, too, with the nurses' suggestions as well as her own and Mr. Burnett's, a considerable library had been organized, and each week the district superintendents obtained books and magazines for the use of their nurses. In 1917, this circulating library, which had been in the hands of the Division of Social Service, was transferred to the central library of the Department, which Dr. Hastings had fostered. Miss Dyke felt, however, that this valuable resource was "not yet being used to the fullest extent", and, at the time of the transfer, she undertook to increase its usefulness by adopting a plan for crediting each nurse with the reading she had done. This, she hoped, would ensure that the nursing staff kept up-to-date with developments in their profession.

Further, Miss Dyke having herself had the stimulus of attending conferences and conventions that related to the expanding concerns of the field of public health nursing, encouraged similar contacts for her nurses. In June 1917, in her report to Dr. Hastings, she expressed appreciation of leave of absence for herself and four nurses to attend the Convention of the Canadian National Association of Trained Nurses in Montreal. "I was glad to have so many of our staff in touch with nursing organization work", she wrote and added that papers by two of her staff had been well received. Both papers, later published in *The Canadian Nurse*, dealt with subjects in which the two women had acquired expertise: Mary Stirritt on *Child Placing*, a field that was new to Canadian nurses, and Enid Forsythe on *Child Welfare Clinics*, 19 of which existed in Toronto at the time.[9] Earlier in the year three nurses had attended some sessions of the Annual Meeting of the Ontario Education Association. Those who enjoyed these privileges were from the executive ranks, however; a fact that probably influenced the decision taken in 1919 to create the Council of Public Health Nurses, opening the way to wider selection for attendance at conventions.

Meanwhile the educational possibilities of the work of the Division of Public Health Nursing were being tapped by outside organizations. Since 1915 the Victorian Order had been sending its student nurses for a week's orientation to public health nursing in the city and in 1916 the privilege was extended to hospital student nurses. Also, the University Department of Social Service experimented with sending a medical social service student for field experience with Department of Public Health nurses. Then, in 1918, on the advice of Jean Gunn, Superintendent of Nurses at the Toronto General Hospital, Kathleen Russell, who had graduated from Dalhousie University and the Toronto General Hospital Training School for Nurses, was awarded a scholarship for the University medical social service course. Then in May 1919, she was appointed to the nursing staff of the

Department of Public Health for experience in public health work.[10] A year later Miss Russell was added to the staff of the University Department of Social Service,[11] and in 1920, when the University, with support from the Ontario Red Cross Society, established a department of public health nursing, Miss Russell was appointed as the Director.

The Red Cross Society had assumed the cost of this venture for a period of three years "as a demonstration and experiment" and, to encourage enrolment, offered 10 scholarships valued at $350, in each of the first two years. In October 1919, The Canadian Red Cross Society wrote to Sir Robert Falconer, President of the University of Toronto to find out whether the University was interested in establishing a course in Public Health Nursing .... In March 1920, Col. Geo. C. Nasmith, Executive Chairman of the Ontario Division of the Red Cross, made a definite offer and enclosed a suggested curriculum .... The Red Cross, he said, did not write to prevent or forestall the extension of public health work under provincial and municipal authorities, nor in any way interfere with the proper duties of the university as a teaching body for the province and for this reason the offer covered a limited period .... The idea of the Red Cross was to make it possible for a community to experience the value of the public health nurses, believing that the demonstration of the nurse's value would result in the establishment of a permanent nursing service under municipal, township or provincial authorities. The Society suggested further, that the Director be a graduate nurse with university public health education. President Falconer replied 15 May that the Senate and the University had unanimously accepted the offer. In 1923 the University assumed responsibility for the Department of Public Health Nursing.[12] Admission to the new Department, forerunner of the University of Toronto Faculty of Nursing, was to be restricted to 50 students who were either graduate nurses on the provincial register, or members of the Canadian National Association of Trained Nurses resident in Ontario. The educational qualification was either matriculation for admission to a Canadian University or a Teachers' Certificate of at least second class grade. The first session of the new Department extended over an eight-month period beginning 28 September 1920, the curriculum including courses provided by the University

114

departments of Hygiene, Medicine, Psychiatry, Household Science and Social Service to supplement the work in Public Health Nursing.[13]

As from 1921, a diploma certifying completion of this one-year course was made obligatory for appointment to the nursing staff of the Toronto Department of Public Health.[14] Miss Dyke triumphed in this decision which guaranteed more adequate preparation for Toronto's public health nurses. Moreover, she had been closely associated with the development of the University Department. Her name is listed among members of the advisory committee, and in January 1921 one of her nurses, Miss E.A. Haines, who had had teaching experience and post graduate training at Columbia University was granted leave to work with Miss Russell as supervisor of "the practical work of the students". Later, two more of her most outstanding nurses, Florence Emory and Mary Millman joined the staff of the School of Nursing. This name adopted in 1933 has since been changed to the Faculty of Nursing. They both served as faculty members for long periods.

Furthermore, in the beginning, students of the new University Department spent 15 hours a week over a period of seven weeks in observation and practice with the city's Division of Public Health Nursing, ensuring a continuing relationship between the two entities. There was provision, also, for occasional students who might register in *two* or *three* subjects: Medicine, Hygiene and Preventive Medicine, and Principles of Teaching. In the fall of 1920, Miss Russell reported that of the 70 'occasionals' who were registered, 47 were members of the nursing staff of the Toronto Department of Public Health. "These," she wrote, "are nurses for whom special training was not available in the past and who are anxious to obtain any help to fit them for their work."[15]

At the same time, hospital training schools in the city were taking further steps to provide public health nursing experience for their student nurses. In October 1923, Dr. Hastings informed the Board of Health that the hospital training schools of the city were sending senior student nurses in groups averaging 17 in number for a period of eight weeks each. As a result student nurses were gathering impressions of public health that would bring the point of view of the homes to their training schools. It was experience, he told the Board, that would help to counteract the tendency of hospitals to treat the patient without reference to his or her environment.

Education for public health nursing became a subject of continuing discussion and experimentation. It had soon been recognized that a one-year course was insufficient post-graduate education to prepare a candidate for the profession, and the program offered by the University Department of Public Health Nursing was extended to meet the need more adequately. In 1926, a four-year course planned in cooperation with the School of Nursing of the Toronto General Hospital was introduced. The first year spent in study at the University, included foundation work in science, and the second and third years were spent in the Hospital's School, with arrangements for the students to earn that School's diploma in hospital nursing. For their fourth year they returned to the University for study of organized public health nursing. As far as possible the four years were planned to follow consecutively, although in reality, the plan involved two courses dependent the one upon the other. Miss Russell kept in touch with courses offered in other schools, both in Canada and in other countries, and her insightful leadership brought world-wide recognition to the University of Toronto school. The course, as altered from time to time, remained a necessary qualification for admission to the Nursing Division of the Toronto Department of Public Health.

To supplement opportunities for training in Toronto, Miss Dyke took pains to ensure that the most promising of her staff would have periods of further education outside the country to broaden their outlook and improve their skills. In Florence Emory, who had joined the staff in 1915, she recognized one of the ablest of the group. Thus in 1923, Miss Emory was awarded a fellowship by the American Child Health Association and given leave for study at Simmons College in Boston with lectures also at the Massachusetts Institute of Technology. It was an experience that served her well for, shortly after her return, she was appointed to Miss Russell's staff in the University Department of Nursing where she spent many fruitful years. One of her achievements was the writing of *Public Health Nursing in Canada*, a comprehensive study of the subject, first published in 1949 and for decades used as a text-book in schools of nursing across the country. Now, in long retrospect, Miss Emory both speaks and writes appreciatively of Miss Dyke's influence on the development of public health nursing in Canada and abroad. Another nurse who enjoyed similar privilege of study outside Canada was Nora Moore, who succeeded Miss Dyke as Director of the Division of Public Health Nursing. She went to England for study at Bedford College of the University of London. Ethel Cryderman, later Superintendent of the Victorian Order of Nurses, also had leave from the Department of Public Health for study in England. Alice Thomson, who edited the Division's 'Red Books' on the expectant mother and infant care and became recognized as an authority on child welfare nursing, went to New York for a period of study at Columbia University. Emma de V. Clarke, who was assigned special responsibilities in psychiatric nursing, was granted a Rockefeller Fellowship for study at Smith College, in Northampton, Massachusetts, and Miss B.A. Moss took advantage of an opportunity for study at Teacher's College, Columbia University. Others had shorter periods away, for example, Mary Irene Foy, who attended the Summer Session of Cleveland School of Nursing in 1916.[17]

In Miss Dyke's opinion, the value of such experience was beyond question, and she favoured a policy that would make it a condition of promotion to an executive position in the Division. In her zeal, however, she overlooked the fact that some of her nurses just as firmly believed that the test of years of work in the Division was more reliable than study abroad as a criterion for promotion to a higher post. Not surprisingly then, Miss Dyke was dismayed when Jessie Woods, a long-term member of the staff, resigned rather than accept a fellowship for study in the field of maternal care. Miss Woods had joined the staff as a measles nurse during the epidemic in the fall of 1912. She had acquired extensive experience under the 'generalized plan' of nursing that Miss Dyke herself had introduced and had been appointed Supervisor of Child and Maternal Service. In Miss Woods' opinion, Miss Dyke's insistence on further training smacked of disloyalty to the pioneer nurses of the Division and lack of appreciation of their work. It was not the first time Miss Dyke had had to consider the value of post-graduate study as compared with experience in the field.

117

Both Dr. Hastings and Nora Moore supported Miss Woods in her rejection of the fellowship, but Miss Dyke pressed her opinion until the disagreement reached a crisis. Dr. Hastings, thoroughly exasperated, ruled that all such educational privileges be withdrawn. The conclusion of the dispute was that Miss Woods withdrew her resignation and returned to the staff of one of the district offices.[18] Miss Dyke described the decision as "a retardation of staff education". Reluctant to criticise Dr. Hastings, however, she attributed the action to his declining years when he was "far from well", but she seemed oblivious to her own single-mindedness in the matter.

Chapter Seven

Arousing Public Awareness

Marshalling the resources of the community: "it is the team... that wins the game".

Rewarding and fruitful as were Miss Dyke's educational achievements in and for the Division for which she was responsible in the Toronto Department of Public Health, she needed and sought the reinforcement that came from participation in nurses' organizations which, at both provincial and national levels, were concerned to improve the educational standards of the profession in general. It was an objective that the Graduate Nurses' Association of Ontario (GNAO) had written into its first Constitution in April 1905. At the same time, the Association authorized an approach to Dr. James Loudon, President of the University of Toronto, to request that the University consider extending its curriculum to include training in nursing.[1] When the Canadian Society of Superintendents of Training Schools for Nurses was founded in 1907, discussion of the subject was opened up at a national level, and the cause was taken up by the Canadian National Association of Trained Nurses (CNATN) which was organized by a group of alumnae in 1908.[2]

By 1914 all the provinces, with the exception of Prince Edward Island, had formed provincial associations which had become members of the national body, and the fourth general meeting of the CNATN, held that year in Halifax, received the report of a committee that recommended the establishment of nurse training schools or colleges in connection with the educational system of each province, institutions separate from hospitals, that would be concerned with the education of the nurse and not, as under the existing system, with "lessening of the cost of nursing in the hospitals". Hospitals would continue to give the practical training, but it would be in the form of a regular course supervised by experienced nurse teachers. Each school would have a staff of lecturers and offer a pass course with a certificate at the end. Students who completed the proposed course would be eligible for additional training in a particular area – district and public health nursing, social service work, hospital administration or the training of teachers of nurses – and on completion of the work, receive a special certificate. To implement its recommendations, the committee suggested that each provincial association appoint a committee to work out a program along these lines and urge the educational authorities to include nurse training in any plan for vocational training they might adopt. Further, no doubt because the report was ruthlessly critical of existing training, the meeting was admonished to consider the whole matter calmly, "not from a personal standpoint, but from that of *Summum Bonum*".[3]

Miss Dyke moved that the report be discussed in detail, explaining that she thought many of those present would endorse parts of it, but her contribution to the discussion was tentative. She recalled 'a long talk' she had recently had with Dr. Cabot who had maintained that the existing three-year course unfitted a nurse for successful work because "the powers of initiative were repressed in her". She thought that his criticism would not apply to "50 per cent of the schools", but added, ". . . still he had stated and printed in writing that the training of the nurse teaches her to follow the lead and crushes all power of initiative". Jean Gunn, Superintendent of Nurses in the Toronto General Hospital, who was chairing the discussion, retorted that, despite this critical stance, Dr. Cabot "moved heaven and earth to get trained nurses as his social workers".

Miss Dyke's intervention had added nothing to the substance of the discussion. By referring to conversation with so renowned an individual as Richard Cabot, who was a member of the Harvard Faculty and, at the time, chief of the medical staff of Massachusetts General Hospital in Bos-

120

ton, she hoped his comment might strengthen the committee's criticism of current teaching practice. In any case, the Association finally decided to appoint a national convener who would receive reports from provincial committees whose members would form a representative national committee to carry forward the work of the special committee.

Progress measured in the terms suggested by the special committee was slow. Not for many years were educational standards for training schools for nurses guaranteed by provincial authorities. Under these circumstances, the provincial nurses' associations accepted responsibility for setting standards, but, since these were not imposed by law, standards of admission varied from hospital to hospital. For Miss Dyke, concerned with the preparation of public health nurses, this variation in standards posed a particular problem, and she advised municipalities in Ontario to require that public health nurses whom they employed be graduates of hospital schools that recognized the criteria set by their provincial Graduate Nurses' Association.[4] Only graduates of such hospitals were eligible for membership in the GNAO and, when the University of Toronto Department of Public Health Nursing was formed in 1920, candidates for admission were required either to be members of the GNAO or to have equivalent status.[5]

At that same general meeting of the CNATN in 1914, as convener of a committee appointed a year earlier to report on the advisability of forming an association of public health and social service nurses,[6] Miss Dyke presented the findings which she described as "difficulties met rather than work done". Appointment of members of the committee had been left to her, and she had had only moderate success in securing an active representative from each province. However, the committee had collected from towns and cities in several provinces information about agencies and institutions that employed nurses in various types of public health work: tuberculosis, pre-natal and child welfare, school inspection, home instruction, visiting nurse services and social relief work. The results were meagre, however, as were the responses to enquiries sent to England, New Zealand and the United States. The Committee had concluded, therefore, that public health nursing was not yet sufficiently established to justify the formation of a special association. Instead, it was suggested that CNATN form a standing committee on public health and social service composed of a convener appointed by the National Association and one representative appointed by each provincial association. Members of this committee would be expected to report local progress in public health and social service nursing at regular meetings of their provincial associations and mail their reports promptly to the national convener. In turn the convener would forward copies of the reports to other provincial representatives and summarize them for the annual meeting of the National Association. Further it was recommended that either a national magazine or a section of the existing magazine be devoted to public health and social service nursing.[7]

In the following year, Mary Ard Mackenzie, Chief Superintendent of the Victorian Order of Nurses, who had chaired the special committee on nursing education, wrote a series of articles denouncing the quality of nursing education. Training schools were exploiting their students "in order to secure cheap nursing in hospitals", she declared, and the profession was losing desirable candidates. Such training as they were given prepared students for institutional nursing only. Even private nursing was neglected, and the broader fields of public health and district nursing, social service and hospital administration were ignored. Published in *The Public Health Journal*, these articles reached a wider audience than was available through *The Canadian Nurse.*[8] Miss Dyke must have been aware of them, but she seems to have ignored them or, at any rate, not to have referred to them publicly. Her consuming concern was to ensure the provision of training in public health nursing, and, if hospital schools conformed to GNAO standards of admission, it would appear that she was willing to accept the training they offered as a basis for further education in public health. Moreover, in her opinion, not less urgent than educational provision for public health and fundamental to achieving that end, was the task of arousing public awareness of the crucial role of the public health nurse in the prevention of disease and the promotion of health. This was a conviction that was fully shared by Dr. Hastings. He continued to be proud of the progress that had been made in his own department but was dismayed that it received so little recognition in Toronto.[9]

Miss Dyke herself, with the bulwark of Dr. Hastings' support, missed no opportunity "to spread the gospel". She welcomed invitations to speak to groups such as the Women's Institute of Clarkson, Ontario, and the Alumnae Association of the University of Toronto Department of Social Service. Referring to the latter talk, given early in March 1917, she wrote, "The point I endeavoured to make was that the problems which the nurses meet in their daily work require that the public health nurse shall not be limited in her opportunity by any traditional concept of a nurse's function". In the fall of 1917 before the Conference of Charities and Correction, she read a paper on "The Organization of Public Health Nursing" in which she summed up the requisites for the organization of public health nursing in four points drawn from the Toronto experience:

> The nurse should be a graduate of a recognized training school; the smallest staff should have one member responsible for the organization of their work; close cooperation should be maintained with other welfare organizations, but complete identification avoided; and in order to secure this last point, the public health nurse should be responsible to the Medical Officer of Health.

The paper ended with a terse statement of her basic conviction: "Prevention of disease is not the least part of a social programme".[10]

Florence Emory's comment that Miss Dyke was keen on cooperation with other civic agencies was seldom more evident than in her concept of the contribution of the public health nurse to "a constructive social programme". In an article published in *The Canadian Nurse* in December 1919, she described a strategy for "team play for health", with the public health nurse in the role of a teacher, or more accurately a strategist, whether in the home, the school or the factory. "The nurse who works *for* others is easily found," she wrote. "... the nurse who works *with* others is the one with a wider influence for health." She advised the inexperienced public health nurse to list "the people who are, or should be, interested in the health of the baby, school child or adult ..." and to compile "a list of the individuals and organizations interested in the health of the community,

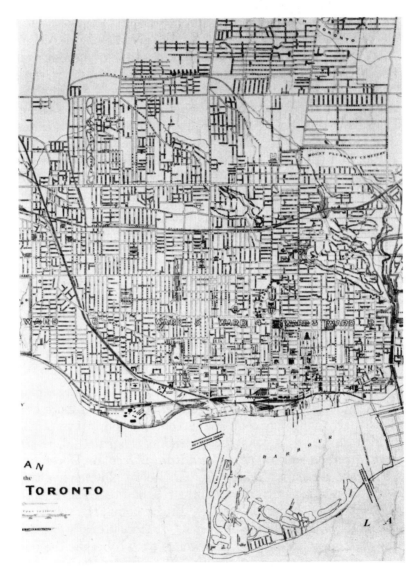

City of Toronto Map of 1912

recording also the reason for their interest and the possible influence they might exert".

> The public health nurse must ... learn to study the background and point of view of those she serves, and must also study the point of view of those individuals or organizations who are, or might become, interested in the health of the community.

In the case of children, parents would come first in the list, because they wanted their children to be healthy and were prepared to sacrifice for them. Unmoved by, perhaps unaware of, the implied condescension, she added that their interest might be unintelligent, but the nurse could build upon the good in it. At the same time, she warned against making the school child "the critic or advisor in home affairs, which are the responsibility of father and mother".

> The most tragic thing that can happen to any child is to lose respect for his father and mother, and the easiest way to antagonise a mother or father is to make the child respect the opinion of teacher or nurse more than that of the home.

Better the school nurse find a way of reaching the home directly through a parents' association or by meeting parents individually, than to foster antagonism between parents and their children. Often times the Clergy, minister or priest of the denomination with which the family was identified, would support the nurse in handling difficult situations.

Employers, because of their interest in the efficiency of their employees, were "a strong factor in the health of the community". The public health nurse should raise with them questions about the age of beginners in their employ, overtime work for adolescents, ventilation, and lack of clean, well placed washrooms. Low standards in an industry should be investigated by the Department of Labour, and the practices of an industry with good standards might be made "a matter of community pride".

Also, the public health nurse should find allies in Municipal Boards: councils, boards of health and education, and all official bodies. If such people did not understand the health needs of the community, those needs had probably not been presented to them in language that compelled their interest. Women's organizations, the Red Cross Society and other public opinion forming groups such as churches and political associations, could help to promote the health of the community. She believed, however, that it would be 'fatal' for the public health nurse to become identified in the minds of the public with any one religious or political group and added that similar difficulties might arise with labour unions and employers' associations.

Finally, there were the Medical Agencies – among whom coordination was often lacking. For good team play, the players must know each other and the part each might play. Miss Dyke was hopeful that inclusion of public health nursing in the hospital educational course with student nurses going to public health services for field work would foster mutual understanding. "The critical interest of the training schools will be good for us", she wrote. Furthermore, public health nurses might "bring a new vision into the hospital wards".

In all situations, however, a safe rule was never to do anything that another could do better, for example, "if a hospital outdoor department is equipped to give special treatment, why establish a school clinic"? Also, for effective team work, there must be a leader, a role that rested in the municipal, provincial and federal departments of health. To be equal to her responsibility, the public health nurse, whose hospital training had been inadequate to the demands of her work should be spending part of her salary on "books and magazines and perhaps post-graduate courses". In conclusion she stressed the importance of access to statistical tables of morbidity and mortality which indicated the measure of success or failure of public health work from year to year. Then she clinched her argument with the aphorism, "... it is the team, not the individual, that wins the game".[11]

Meanwhile, the Public Health Committee of the CNATN, which Miss Dyke convened, had worked through its task of assembling responses to questionnaires sent to provincial representatives. There were reports from the Victorian Order, municipal boards of health, a provincial board of health, boards of education, hospitals, the Metropolitan Life Insurance Company, Women's Institutes and other voluntary organizations. They provided current information

126

about visiting nursing, instructive tuberculosis and child welfare nursing, sanitary inspection, medical social service in hospitals and school nursing, but none on industrial nursing. As a result of this exercise, in May 1917, Miss Dyke submitted recommendations to members of the Committee, among them one that advocated the organizing of a public health section with its own officers and representation on the Council of the CNATN. Her suggestion was rejected by a vote of four to three. Undaunted, however, she directed the attention of the CNATN to the likelihood of a substantial increase in the demand for preventive nursing in the post-war period of reconstruction which should be kept in mind in planning a standard curriculum for schools of nurses. Meanwhile, it would be necessary to provide the best nurses available, those "with a thorough knowledge of nursing practice and health laws and high ideals of service". To press home the urgency of the situation, she quoted a recommendation that had been submitted by "a pioneer Canadian public health nurse".

> That superintendents of training schools be urged to draw the attention of their prospective graduates to this new field of nursing activity, a field which, being educational in character, requires a type of nurse in whom teaching ability is pronounced, combined with a love of children and the missionary spirit, and, as this field of work is destined to be much more greatly developed in future, ... superintendents of nurses should urge the nurses with the qualifications mentioned to especially fit themselves to enter this field.[12]

Again in 1918, speaking for her Committee at the annual meeting of the CNATN, Miss Dyke reminded the Association of the inadequacy of facilities for training public health nursing and urged the importance of strengthening the public health nursing group "in every way possible". Discussion of her report was deferred,[13] but within a year, the war had come to an end and the tasks of reconstruction were no longer a distant goal. At the General Meeting of the CNATN held in Vancouver in July 1919, Miss Gunn, who was President of the Association, made a stirring plea for a broadened approach to the field of nursing. The previous five years had brought many changes in the nation as a whole and to nursing in particular. "We are assuming a great many more responsibilities than we had during the period of the war." She also stressed the growing interest in public health work, "one of the very best outcomes of the war".[14]

It was a favourable atmosphere for the creation of a public health section within the Association, and Miss Dyke was appointed convener of a committee to submit a plan of organization at the next annual meeting. A letter that she wrote to members of her committee on 27 August 1919 shows that for her a crucial question was whether officers of the section would be appointed by the Executive Committee of the CNATN or elected by members of the Association who were actively engaged in public health work. She preferred the latter, her thinly disguised aim being to ensure a degree of autonomy for the section. The matter was discussed at meetings of the CNATN Executive in February and April of 1920. Then at the Annual Meeting of the Association in July, Miss Dyke presided at a round table conference on public health subjects, and a resolution that a public health section be formed was carried unanimously.[15]

For the first year of the Section's existence, Miss Dyke was chairman, but in the years that followed she is not again listed as an officer. Doubtless that mattered to her less than that at last public health nursing had become one of the foremost concerns of the CNATN. Moreover, she continued to participate in the work of the Section and to influence decisions of policy. In June 1921, at the Tenth General Meeting of the National Association held in Quebec, she spoke on "Generalized Public Health", describing the pioneering experience with that concept in her own Division in the Toronto Department of Public Health.[16]

Meanwhile she had become involved in another national development in nursing service. After the war the Canadian Red Cross Society had taken steps to amend its Charter in conformity with the decision of the International Red Cross to change its policy and program to include peacetime service for "the improvement of health, the prevention of disease and the mitigation of suffering". This new emphasis would require the creation of a national nursing service, and it was evident that the CNATN should have a voice in the process. In June 1919, therefore, the Board of Directors of the CNATN appointed a committee of which Miss Dyke was a member "to draft a policy for a nursing service under the auspices of the Red Cross".[17] Subsequent action on the part of the Convention held in July in Vancouver led to the appointment of a fully representative committee and a sub-committee of which Miss Gunn and Miss Dyke were chairman and secretary, respectively.

The Committee acted promptly, and even before the amendment of the Red Cross Act of Incorporation had been completed, the CNATN had invited the Society to cooperate in a broad-ranging program to improve and expand nursing service throughout the country. The most important recommendations were: i. that a national registration of nurses be set up to cope with emergencies; ii. that more women be encouraged to take professional nurses' training; iii. that standards of training be improved, the claim of nurses being brought to the attention of universities; and iv. that training be provided for nurses' aides. Consultation with the Red Cross Society, encouraged that CNATN Committee but, when the Central Council of the Society met in September, it decided to move out on broader lines and form an Emergency Medical and Nursing Service that would include doctors, voluntary workers and semi-trained as well as professional nurses. Further, the Council would form a committee on which representatives of interested organizations would serve. There would be provision for registration of nurses, but more important, the Council adopted the suggestion that universities be encouraged to introduce nursing education.[18] In fact, when Miss Dyke reported on the work of the Committee on National Nursing Service in November, 1919, the Red Cross Society had already written to all of the provincial universities and had notified its provincial branches "to be prepared to take the matter up with their own universities".[19]

The Central Council of the Red Cross Society referred further planning of the Medical and Nursing Service to the central executive which in turn appointed Miss Dyke to be associated with General Ryerson in outlining organization and policy for the proposed Service. Gen. Stirling Ryerson was responsible for reorganization of the Canadian Red Cross Society after the first World War. In her report to the CNATN, Miss Dyke stated that development of a national nursing service would follow the formation of the special committee to be appointed by the Red Cross Society. Further, she emphasized that successful cooperation between the Society and the CNATN would require that representative nurses should be named to committees appointed by the Red Cross to deal with the subject. The CNATN Committee on a National Nursing Service was continued until 1921 by which time the Red Cross Society had taken up the work and was closely in touch with all of the provincial nurses' associations and through them with the CNATN.[20]

Miss Dyke continued to participate actively in the CNATN, which in 1924 was renamed the Canadian Nurses' Association (CNA). During 1926-27, as councillor for the Registered Nurses Association of Ontario, she was a member of the Executive Committee,[21] and in that capacity, in 1927, she spoke to the Public Health Section about trends in public health nursing in the Province. For her it was another opportunity to expound her conception of the role of the public health nurse and her need of special training, an exercise that she undertook with evangelical zeal. Without reports from district councillors, she spoke for herself using the pronoun, 'I'.

Once again the theme of 'team play for health' came through strongly, but this time she talked about consciousness of a common task. She noted efforts on the part of public health nurses to enlist workers from other professions and to draw upon their experience in behalf of families in need of their skills. She gave examples of cooperation with teachers, social workers and occupational therapists and cited the cooperation of household science and social workers with nurses in guiding the visiting housekeeper service in Toronto. She mentioned also a recent luncheon in Toronto when the formation of a council of health agencies under the chairmanship of the president of the Academy of Medicine had been proposed.

In this development she saw a parallel to "the tendency to combine all nursing services required by the family in the person of one individual nurse", in other words, the principle of generalized nursing with which she was identified as a result of her by then well-known achievement in Toronto. She reminded her audience that such cooperation would conserve time and energy and unify the efforts of physicians and others interested in a family. She believed, moreover, that it was "in harmony with the natural impulses of women doing public health work". In contrast to the physician, presumably a man, whose interest lay in a particular field of medicine, the woman's response was "to the patient, the family ... never to a disease". Individuals and their human relationships were paramount for the nurse: "Disease present or as a future possibility interests her only as it may affect the people for whom she is responsible".

The chief thrust of the paper, however, had to do with the education of public health nurses. By that time, largely as a result of 'the conscious demand' of pioneer public health nurses, two universities in the province (the University of Toronto and the University of Western Ontario) had introduced special courses in public health. Such efforts, she thought, should be recorded before the women who made them were forgotten. Scholarships had been offered by hospital trustees, the Board of the V.O.N., the Ontario Red Cross and nurses' associations. Nevertheless, a majority of nurses in public health work were still "facing new tasks with the handicaps of the early pioneers". Only 297 nurses had graduated from the university departments in the previous seven years; only two public health organizations in Ontario required special training for their nurses *before* appointment, and there was no provision for special training *after* appointment. She could see no hope of convincing employers, however, until private physicians accepted the need of special training for public health nurses. Every student graduating from the Toronto School of Medicine spent a month in the City's Department of Public Health, and the nurses of the Department must "enlighten these physicians of the future". Imagine them escaping Miss Dyke's influence, let alone that of her nurses!

A trend that she noted with satisfaction was that superintendents of hospital training schools who were in touch with the public health movement were questioning whether their "standard of curriculum" gave adequate foundation training for the public health nurse. It was in the previous year that the University of Toronto and the Toronto General Hospital had introduced the four-year course in which the University would teach selected subjects in the humanities, sciences and public health in the first and fourth years with the Hospital giving basic nursing content in the two intervening years. Miss Dyke made no reference to the leadership of Kathleen Russell and her colleagues in working out this new course with the University and the Hospital, but commented somewhat obscurely that it would "demonstrate the value of the hospital experience for students at the outset of their four years' course on the basis of their personal qualifications for public health work".

Returning to the theme of health teaching, she ended her talk by suggesting that the time might come in Ontario when Florence Nightingale's terms, 'sick nursing' and 'health nursing' might supplant such titles as hospital nursing and public health nursing. Such a step, she thought, would better describe "the elements present in varying degrees in the work of all nurses, whether ... employed in hospitals and in the home to care for the sick or as medical social workers and health visitors to maintain health".[22]

Miss Dyke's last opportunity to influence CNA thinking about public health nursing and appropriate preparation for it occurred in June 1932, when she gave a paper on the implications of the Weir Survey of Nursing Education at the Public Health Nursing Section during the General Meeting of the Association. The Report was a landmark in the history of the nursing profession in Canada, the result of a detailed survey sponsored jointly by the Canadian Medical Association and the Canadian Nurses' Association and carried out under the direction of Dr. George M. Weir, Professor of Education and Head of the Department of Education at the University of British Columbia. The enquiry had tackled the question of selection, allocation and grading of training schools for nurses and the costs involved. It had elicited information about admission and graduation requirements, the size of classes and the content of curriculum. It investigated economic and other factors affecting the professional status of nurses, their income and their opportunities for growth through recreation, study and travel, and causes of the current unemployment among nurses.[23]

For Eunice Dyke, "the clear message of the Survey" was that Canada had "permitted the hospital rather than the community to dominate the nursing profession ...". Henceforth public health nurses must accept a burden of responsibility for interpreting the needs of the community to the rest of the profession. She selected two emphases of the

Report: First, that nursing schools should be financed by and responsible to the community, and second, that nursing forces should be organized on a basis that would be acceptable to the public and to the nurses themselves. Then she talked about how public health nurses might contribute to these ends.

In the first place, if existing dissatisfaction with nursing services were to be overcome, the nursing profession must set about convincing legislative bodies that training schools should be independent of hospitals but use selected hospitals for the teaching of basic nursing. Further, public health nurses in their community contacts must explain that existing hospital schools were "one cause of their limitations". Secondly, public health nurses, nurse instructors and head nurses must together study the method and content of instruction in the hospital schools in order to work toward a change of emphasis in the selection of students and in teaching programs.

To achieve a sense of unity among nursing forces, she suggested that local associations bring together representatives of hospitals, private duty and public health nurses in order to encourage group learning. For example, they might discuss whether a student should be taught to bathe an infant on a table or on the knee. Seemingly, a trivial question, it would illustrate how consideration of household equipment and family life should influence the teaching in a hospital school. Or, study of the relation of a patient's family to the hospital might suggest the value of telephone interviews and home visits for teaching purposes. Or again, the hospital course in dietetics might include a demonstration by the dietitian of how best to use the food provided by a relief agency. Also, to stimulate thinking about the organization of community nursing forces, she suggested that local nursing associations debate the topic: "Resolved that branches of the Victorian Order of Nurses should employ a second group of salaried nurses to provide resident nursing care in the homes". She thought that in the Victorian Order there might be the answer to growing demand for "a socialized system of nursing care". Such development of the Victorian Order might be preferable to the district registries suggested by the Survey Report as a solution for problems of distribution and employment of nurses. Moreover, some local nursing associations with representatives of the three groups of nurses (private, hospital and public health) might reduce the problems of distribution and employment to the simplest terms for consideration by the national association.

Her final thrust was that, in stressing the community and its needs, the Survey had presented an objective strong enough to unify the profession and so facilitate cooperation with other professions for the advancement of health standards in Canada. Her paper ended with a tribute to Dr. Weir and the Survey Committee, commending them for the honesty with which they had presented the facts of the existing situation for guidance into the future.[24]

Characteristically didactic, it was, nevertheless, a stimulating presentation of the subject, and, although Miss Dyke had no inkling of the fact, it had been her 'swan song'. A few months later, well before the next general meeting of the Canadian Nurses' Association, her career as Director of the Public Health Nursing Division of the Toronto Department of Public Health had come to a humiliating end.

Chapter Eight

Collapse of a Career

In November 1932, Miss Dyke was dismissed from the post she had filled with distinction for 21 years, but not without protest from colleagues, friends and fellow-citizens. Working with Dr. Hastings, her mentor for almost two decades, she had grown in stature. There had been times of disagreement but she had trusted him implicitly. His successor, Dr. Gordon P. Jackson, knew the Department of Public Health but lacked the insight and administrative capacity of his predecessor. In the opinion of several former nurses of the Department, he was a small-minded individual, while one of the most distinguished of them, an enthusiastic admirer of Dr. Hastings, declares that the only mistake he ever made was to recommend Dr. Jackson as his successor. "To be sure," she adds, "we nurses knew lots of things that the doctors, even Dr. Hastings, didn't know." A less partisan observer from outside the Department of Public Health who had been aware of Dr. Jackson's competence as a district medical officer, remarks that, in the larger sphere of responsibility for the Department as a whole, he was beyond his depth. He was intimidated by the demands of the Board of Control, often even to the extent of waiving his own convictions. He shrank from sessions when his budget was under review and retreated before strictures that would have been a challenge to Dr. Hastings. Miss Dyke, herself a forceful administrator with a substantial reputation as a public health nurse, not only in Toronto but also throughout Canada and abroad, posed a threat to her new chief. She moved with the assurance, some called it arrogance, of having achieved success. It must have taken pluck, probably fortified by male chauvinism, for Dr. Jackson to fire her.

NURSES PROTEST ACTION OF M.O.H. ON TWO MEMBERS

Ask Explanation for Dismissal of One and Suspension for Miss Dyke

LETTER TO MAYOR

Refer to "Wise and Far-Sighted Leadership" of Dr. Hastings

On behalf of the registered nurses' association of Ontario, a letter of protest asking an explanation for dismissal of one nurse and the suspension of Miss Eunice Dyke from the department of public health was received by Mayor Stewart to-day from Miss Matilda E. Fitzgerald, secretary of the organization. The first nurse's dismissal followed the death of a child on Bay St. last July. Miss Dyke's suspension was announced yesterday.

A letter from Dr. Jackson, accompanying the recommendation for suspension, spoke of disloyalty in the department. Miss Fitzgerald's letter to the mayor follows:

"It is with great regret that we, as a nursing organization have found it necessary to appeal to you, and to the public, in regard to the recent developments in the division of public health nursing.

"For many years the division has had a well-deserved and well-maintained international prestige, which came into being through the wise and far-sighted leadership of the

(Continued on Page Two)

The Toronto Daily Star, *7 October 1932*

When the axe fell, it came as a body blow. Stripped of authority and lacking the sense of shared goals she had had with Dr. Hastings, she retorted in anger.

The opening sally occurred on 15 July 1932. It was alleged that on that day a nurse of the Department of Public Health, through neglect of duty, had been the cause of an infant's death. The nurse was Mary E. Bullick who, that morning, was in the City Hall office of the Nursing Division preparing to take over her duties as Acting Superintendent of the University District while the Superintendent was on vacation. The infant was a pre-mature twin of 1.6 kilos at birth, the child of Mr. and Mrs. Michael Kenny of 750 Bay Street. The baby, now four months old, had been sickly and under the close supervision of the district nurse until, fallen ill with pneumonia, it had been taken to the Hospital for Sick Children. On the evening 14 July, although the child was being given interstitial treatment following blood transfusions, the parents took him home against the advice of the hospital doctor who told them they would ruin its one slim chance of recovery.

At nine o'clock the next morning the nursing division received a call for a doctor to visit the Kenny home because of the critical illness of the baby. Waiting only to obtain a hospital report confirming the seriousness of the child's condition and explaining the needed treatment, Miss Bullick visited the home shortly after 10 o'clock. Finding the baby in need of immediate medical attention, she urged the parents to take it at once to the hospital which was only a block away, but the mother refused. She said she would rather have the child die at home, since the doctor at the hospital had said it could not get better anyway. The University District Medical Health Officer was on vacation, and Miss Bullick warned the parents that there would be some delay in getting a city doctor. To go back to the hospital would be the quickest and most satisfactory way to obtain a doctor's service. However, the father objected and joined his wife in declaring that they would not consent to return the infant to the hospital. At 11 o'clock Miss Bullick telephoned the Hillcrest District office to try to reach the medical health officer of that district who, in the absence of the doctors in charge of both the University and St. Clair districts, was attending to calls from those districts as well as his own. He was not in, but Miss Bullick gave the nurse who was on duty the relevant information. During the noon-hour a neighbour of the Kennys telephoned and Miss Bullick told her that the doctor had been asked to visit and was probably on his way. However, she urged the neighbour to try to persuade the parents to take the child to the hospital, where it could be given proper care. Meanwhile another nurse, who knew the family, agreed to stop on her way off duty for a half-day to see what was being done for the baby but, seeing a car that looked like the doctor's parked in front of the Kenny home, she assumed that the patient was now in his care and did not get in touch with Miss Bullick.

Later enquiry revealed, however, that, when the doctor telephoned the Hillcrest office, the Kenny call had been omitted from the list of calls given him. Inadvertently, the written message had been covered by a parcel that had come from the City Hall, and the nurse to whom Miss Bullick had spoken earlier was out in the field. Fifteen minutes later, the record of the call was found, but attempts to reach the doctor were unsuccessful. Early in the afternoon, Miss Bullick, unaware of this sequence of trial and error, met the doctor at the Jewish Boy's Club in Simcoe Street where he was examining boys who were going to camp. She asked him how he had found the baby, only to be told that he had not heard of the case. Horrified at the delay, she gave him a full account of the circumstances, and as soon as possible, he went to the Kenny home, but the baby had already died.[1]

The matter was raised in the Board of Control on 18 July and referred to the Medical Officer of Health. Dr. Jackson, who had been out of the city from the 15th to the 18th, had not heard about the case but made immediate enquiries and, in his report to the Board on 20 July, he attributed the incident not to heartlessness of the nurses but to error and misjudgment on the part of one or more of them. Nevertheless, he believed that error must be acknowledged, and he assured the Board that steps were being taken to censure and discipline the individuals involved. In fact, he had already written to Miss Bullick, to whom he ascribed major blame, informing her that she would be demoted and transferred, but several members of the Board thought demotion of the nurse was not sufficient penalty and called for her dismissal.[2] To consider the problem further, the Board of Health met on 3 August but decided to leave it in the hands of the Medical Officer of Health. On the following day, Dr. Jackson interviewed Miss Bullick at her home but said nothing about dismissal. Nevertheless, on 20 September, when, at his request, she called at his office, he told her that she was dismissed as from 20 July. Dismayed by this decision, she determined to seek legal advice about a claim for salary which she had not been paid during the two months' suspension, and on 6 October 1932, Miss Dyke went with her to see a lawyer and confirm the facts of the case. On returning to the City Hall, Miss Dyke reported to Dr. Jackson what she had done and was herself suspended.[3]

Later, Miss Dyke was reported as having said that, as a civic employee, she had shown poor judgment in assisting Miss Bullick to secure the full facts of the case for her legal adviser,[4] but plainly she had not anticipated such drastic action on the part of the Medical Officer of Health. Only two years previously, when recovering from her cancer operation and uncertain whether her strength would be equal to the demands of her job, she had consulted Dr. Jackson about the advisability of resigning. He had encouraged her to continue, even going so far as to tell her they could not get along without her. No matter how, after further thought, Miss Dyke may have felt about the visit to the lawyer, she was convinced of the injustice done to Miss Bullick who, during six years on the staff, had proven to be a dependable and competent nurse. When the Kenny baby incident occurred, she had been due for promotion.[5]

Inevitably, the other nurses of the Department of Health were caught up in the controversy, and on 16 August, Miss Dyke called them together to discuss Miss Bullick's suspension. Some of the nurses had collected $150 to help compensate her for loss of salary, and several wrote to Dr. Jackson urging leniency toward her. Then when Mis Dyke's suspension was announced, a number of them were so incensed that they refused to speak to Dr. Jackson in the street.[6] He was thoroughly exasperated and, on that same day he wrote to the Mayor and members of the Board of Control a long letter about the difficulties of maintaining discipline in his Department:

Recent events within my Department and the future

possibilities they may carry with them, make it necessary that I acquaint you with what portends to be the establishment of an intolerable situation. . . . The time has come for a definite assertion of authority, with insistence of allegiance to that authority.

His methods, he feared, might be misunderstood by people who were unacquainted with the difficulty of controlling fifteen divisions whose activities, while necessary to a good health regime, were carried on "with a personnel composed of both sexes in some instances of wide variation socially". Under the circumstances he believed that a routine method of discipline would be ineffective, but he was confident that the Board would uphold his judgment, "provided the judgment is not allowed to become biased through pressure of undue influence emanating from outside the Civic Administration". If he were to be constantly subjected to "the threat of implied power" from without, his administration would be hampered, "with devastating effect on the morale of the Department".[7]

In response, the Mayor assured Dr. Jackson that the administration of the Department of Public Health was entirely in his hands and it was for him to demand to the fullest extent the highest measure of efficiency and loyalty from all members of his staff. Any action that he took would receive the unanimous support of the Board of Control. Further, the Mayor emphasized that influence or interference from outside bodies would not be tolerated.

At first Dr. Jackson refused to make any statement to the press, although he did contend in a conversation with a reporter from *The Globe*, that his letter to the Mayor and the Board of Control had nothing to do with Miss Dyke's suspension. The timing of the two things was merely a coincidence, and he was quoted as having added: "I prefer to keep the reason for suspension to myself".

The newspapers had no scruples about seeking other sources of information, however, and they attacked the injustice done to the two nurses; *The Toronto Daily Star* made it "une cause célèbre". Many were disturbed when they read one nurse's account in that paper:

Dr. Jackson told the nurses that time must not be taken up during office hours to discuss the case, that the suspended nurse had been discharged and that anyone found discussing the case inside or outside the office would also be discharged. The whole affair, he said, must be dropped.

Also, there were protests from the members of the public, both organizations and individuals. As early as 28 July, a letter from Mrs. A.L. Hynes, President of the Local Council of Women, asked the Mayor for an explanation of the action taken in respect to Miss Bullick, but the most forceful pressure of public opinion came during October and November and even in 1933. One of the strongest submissions came on 7 October when the Registered Nurses' Association of Ontario (RNAO) released to the press a letter to the Mayor asking for an explanation of "recent developments in the Division of Public Health Nursing":

> For many years the division has had a well-deserved and well maintained international prestige, which came into being through the wise and far-sighted leadership of the late Dr. C.J.O. Hastings, ably assisted by the director of the division, Miss Eunice Dyke. We feel that a full explanation is due the nursing profession, of which the two nurses now under discipline are honored members.

Enclosed with the letter, signed by Matilda E. Fitzgerald, Secretary of the Association, were two statements, one from Miss Bullick describing the sequence of events on 15 July; the other, a further protest against the dismissal of "a nurse who possesses an excellent record of six years" of service with the Department of Public Health and in regard to whose work and character no question had ever risen before. The RNAO also asked why only one person concerned in "the regrettable incident with the Kenny family" had been selected for special discipline and subsequent dismissal and asked for "a full explanation of the drastic action taken by the Medical Officer of Health in dealing with a nurse who had been the efficient director of the division of public health since its organization 21 years ago".

The Mayor, in acknowledging receipt of the letter, merely advised the Association that Dr. Jackson as Medical Officer of Health was responsible for the administration of the Department. He refused to discuss the RNAO protest with the press except to say that he supported Dr. Jackson and would listen to no representatives from outside concerning the internal administration of the Department.[8]

Members of the City Council, sensitive to public opinion, were divided on the issue. Advocates of an inquiry into the circumstances of Miss Bullick's dismissal were in a minority, and the Mayor ruled the proposal out of order, 17 October 1932. At a joint meeting of the Board of Control and the Board of Health on 20 October, it was decided, however, that "in view of the wide publicity given the case", Dr. Jackson should be called in to answer "certain questions" relating to the subject. Asked whether Miss Bullick had been made a scapegoat for any person or persons, he answered an emphatic, "No!" Nor did he think that she had been treated unjustly. He considered that she had failed in her duty as an experienced departmental nurse in not responding to a request for a physician to attend an emergency case and could not be trusted to perform the required duties satisfactorily. She had therefore been demoted and transferred and later dismissed because, "in view of the wide publicity given the matter", he thought public confidence in the Department would be seriously impaired if she were retained in the service. He admitted that a head of a division of his Department had been under suspicion and explained that her suspension was "a measure of discipline". As Head of the Department, responsible for its work, he felt that he was entitled to the loyalty and cooperation of all its members. Moreover, he contended that the By-laws of the Council gave him authority to mete out discipline. The Board, accepting his claim, took no action in the matter.

The case dragged on. A letter to the Mayor from Godfrey and Corcoran, Barristers, dated 28 October, reviewed the incidents leading to Miss Bullick's dismissal and informed the Mayor that they had advised Miss Bullick that she had been wrongfully dismissed. They believed that she had been treated with harshness and cruelty and "had been done a great wrong". Unless "full and complete reparations" were made and her reputation cleared, she would be compelled to issue a Writ for wrongful dismissal. They wanted to have the case tried at the Jury Sittings of the County Court in December and, unless they received assurance by 10 o'clock on 31 October that the City Solicitor would expedite them in having a speedy trial, a Writ would be issued at once. They assumed, moreover, that no technical obstacles would be thrown in the way of Miss Bullick having her claim adjudicated by a Jury, since she had suffered from the publicity given the matter.[9]

Under the same date the Mayor replied that he did not wish to be understood as agreeing with the statements about the circumstances of Miss Bullick's dismissal which were "considerably at variance with the facts as reported" to him. Further, he stated that the administration of the Department of Public Health was under the Medical Officer of Health who by Civic By-law had authority "to engage, dismiss, demote or promote any employee of the Department". Forthwith, on 1 November, the Writ, Miss Bullick vs. City of Toronto, was issued. Not until the 8th, however, was the lawyers' letter brought to the attention of the Board of Control and referred to the City Solicitor. Already, on 31 October, the City Council had rejected a motion that the Medical Officer of Health confer with Miss Bullick and Miss Dyke with a view to an amicable settlement and the reinstatement of both women.

On that same day, Dr. Jackson notified Miss Dyke that the city no longer required her services and asked for her resignation by the following morning. Her reply, in which she refused to submit her resignation and asked for a judicial investigation in order that her activities in connection with Miss Bullick's dismissal might be fully presented, reached the Board of Control on 2 November, but the Board still declined to take any action. On 7 November, Miss Dyke wrote again asking what had happened to her letter of 31 October and repeating her request for a judicial investigation.

Protests against the action of the Medical Officer of Health in dismissing both Miss Bullick and Miss Dyke had begun to multiply. They came from individuals and from organizations as diverse as the Local Council of Women, the Independent Labour Party, the Women's Liberal Conservative Association, the Junior League, a Ratepayers' Association, and a section of the Movement for a Christian Social Order.[10] A letter from a reader of *The Toronto Daily Star* in Prince's Lake, Ontario, suggested that the key-note of the trouble lay in the filing system of the doctor's office. She could see no reason for the denunciation of Miss Bullick which, compared to the recent release of two men who had murdered a Chinaman because he persisted in claiming payment for meals eaten in his restaurant, led her to conclude that it was not only in Bible times that people "strained at gnats and swallowed camels".[11] Another, from a Toronto nurse critical of Miss Dyke's administration of the Division of Public Health Nursing, was referred to the Medical Officer of Health. Most of the communications asked for a public investigation of the treatment of the two women, and those from organizations, cited resolutions that had been adopted by their members. None of these was acted on on the grounds that discussion was out of order while the Bullick case was before the Courts. However, as time went on it became more difficult to disregard the protests of responsible individuals and organizations in the community.

Alarmed by growing public criticism, on 15 November, the City Council passed a motion that Dr. Jackson be asked to appear before its members to explain his reason or reasons for Miss Dyke's suspension and dismissal. Because she had been a long-time employee of the Department of Public Health and neither they nor citizens in general knew why the Medical Officer of Health had taken such action, they thought he should be called to account. The Minutes record only that Dr. Jackson appeared and stated his reasons. Not all the members were satisfied, however, and a week later it was agreed that, "since the dismissal of Miss Dyke had been brought about by the dismissal of Miss Bullick, all minutes of the Board of Control dealing with the interviews with Dr. Jackson be read in so far as they related to the dismissal of Miss Bullick".

On 23 November, Miss Dyke herself appeared before the Board of Control ostensibly to present the statement that she had submitted previously about her activities in connection with Miss Bullick's dismissal. The Mayor informed her, however, that members of the Board had just been given copies of her statement and that, because of "its voluminous character", discussion would have to be deferred to allow time for them to read it. The Board requested the Medical Officer of Health to respond to her statement, and five days later members of the Board of Health attended a meeting of the Board of Control without Miss Dyke present to hear what Dr. Jackson had to say about the matter.

Dr. Jackson's response, his defence for having dismissed Miss Dyke, was a devastating attack on her character and conduct. He first explained that, although Miss Dyke's statement dealt almost entirely with her activities in reference to Miss Bullick's dismissal, he would avoid discussion of that subject because the case was currently before the courts. He did wish, however, to correct any impression that the Bullick case was the sole reason for Miss Dyke's dismissal. "It was but the culmination of a series of situations extending over the whole period of my administration, in which I . . . was placed in the embarrassing position of mediator either as a result of her indiscretion or failure to realize that she was a subordinate." It was an open secret, he added, that even Dr. Hastings' regime had not been entirely free from her troublesome interference:

Miss Dyke is one of those individuals who never takes "No" from her superior in office without a prolonged argument, and in contrast interprets the slightest interest shown in any of her propositions as acquiesence thereto . . . Her subtle use of adroit or ingenuous phraseologies, often times conveying and implying impressions which cannot be completely substantiated, is well known to those who are familiar with her . . . Her misinterpretation of conversations with a tendency to jump to conclusions is a common fault.

Much of the value of Miss Dyke's capabilities as an organizer and administrator is lost because she persistently permits her personal likes and dislikes to enter into matters . . . her sudden exploitations of certain members of her staff for a time, only to be dropped with the acquiring of a new interest in another, is a source of discontent and disruption within the service. It is to these well-known traits that can be laid much of the reason for . . . the situation in which Miss Dyke finds herself today.

Dr. Jackson then proceeded, paragraph by paragraph, to repudiate Miss Dyke's account of the incidents following Miss Bullick's suspension. Her account of the meeting of her staff that she had called on 16 August was a special target of his criticism. From "six executive members of the staff" he had obtained signed statements of opinion of what had happened. One of these charged that, with Miss Dyke leading the discussion, "Those who were of the opinion that Miss Bullick had done no wrong were apparently encouraged to speak; those who held contrary opinions were apparently discouraged". Also, although the remarks she made were not direct statements, they gave the impression that Dr. Jackson was in the wrong. Another had written, "My first reaction was that I really had no business there, that it was a matter to be handled by the Director alone ... My second reaction was one of astonishment that the Director, who, expecting loyalty from us, should display even in so subtle a way, such disloyalty to her Medical Officer."

He also drew upon excerpts from Miss Dyke's journal, without explaining how he had got access to them except to say that they were taken "from the original stenographic records". These, he implied, indicated that, behind the scenes, she had been responsible for the protest from the RNAO in October. A note in the diary stated that she had seen the President and learned that the Association was aware of what had happened. Then, at a later date, she had written, "I understand that some definite action will be taken on Friday to bring the three nursing organizations together on the matter of Miss Bullick". In this connection it is interesting that the then president of the RNAO, who vividly recalls the meeting that endorsed the statement sent to Mayor Stewart with a copy to *The Toronto Daily Star*, says emphatically that it was she who initiated the action and that Miss Dyke had nothing at all to do with it.

To substantiate his charges of unrest in the Nursing Division caused by Miss Dyke's autocratic attitude, Dr. Jackson added:

> About two years' [sic] ago, I was called into conference with the Director of Public Health Nursing, University of Toronto, and she reported that cooperation between her Department and my Nursing Division was becoming impossible, because of the dictatorial and interfering activities of Miss Dyke with her students, many of whom take their field work in our Division.

Among Kathleen Russell's papers there is no record of this encounter, but granted it may have happened, Dr. Jackson had been less than honest with Miss Dyke when in 1930, following her long illness, she had consulted him about the wisdom of continuing in her post. Moreover, it was inevitable that two such strong-minded women as Miss Russell and

Miss Dyke would clash from time to time, but Florence Emory, who worked closely with both of them, says that, while they undoubtedly irritated one another, their common goals and mutual respect remained unassailed. Miss Emory also recalls that Miss Russell wholeheartedly supported Miss Dyke's defence of Miss Bullick.

Dr. Jackson's most damaging accusation, however, grew out of a conversation he had had with Miss Dyke when she criticised Dr. Robb, the District Medical Health Officer involved in the case, for not having checked with his office earlier in the day about calls that awaited his attention. She contended that had he telephoned earlier, the nurse who had taken Miss Bullick's message about the Kenny child would still have been in the office. Miss Dyke implied that Dr. Robb was practising medicine on the side and, in any case, was more interested in real estate deals than in keeping in touch with his office. Dr. Jackson had questioned Dr. Robb about the charges Miss Dyke made and he quoted Dr. Robb's response, using the man's own words as nearly as he could remember them:

> I have not made a five cent piece in outside practice in over a year and a half, and my interest in real estate deals consists in owning my own house and the one next door, where I go to collect the rent once a month.

To clinch the matter, Dr. Jackson added, "I know for a fact that Dr. Robb does not even display a sign on his door". He had failed to recognize that Miss Dyke, anxious to defend Miss Bullick and doubtless to justify her own actions, had spoken in anger and frustration. In a flare of temper, she had resorted to insinuations that she would have found it difficult to defend.

Dr. Jackson's final comment was that he had been aware of the turmoil that would follow his dismissal of Miss Dyke. "But," he added, "I could no longer delay definite action as the situation had become intolerable." When he finished speaking, the Board of Control ruled that copies of his statement and of Miss Dyke's letter should be sent to all members of City Council, and the Mayor promised that, when the Bullick case was out of Court, the Medical Officer of Health would be given opportunity to explain the circumstances of the dismissal of the two nurses.[12]

147

In due course the case of Mary E. Bullick vs The Corporation of the City of Toronto had come before His Honour Judge O'Connell of the County Court of the County of York. Evidence in the case had occupied "upwards of two days", and at the end of a detailed review of events, the Judge ruled that, while it was possible that there had been some lapse of judgment on Miss Bullick's part and she might have pursued a better course, the most that could be said was that "it had been an honest lapse of judgment". Moreover, he believed that there were factors in the case of which, if Dr. Jackson had been aware, he would not even have demoted her. Finally, he found that there had been no just cause for her dismissal. Questions of law arising from by-laws and acts relevant to the case he reserved for further consideration. This verdict was particularly disturbing for members of the City Council, and on 13 December, they asked that Minutes of the Board of Control recounting interviews with Dr. Jackson on the subject be read in full. This done, with the judgment in mind, a motion recommending reappointment of Miss Bullick passed by a majority of 12 votes. Further consideration of the motion after the noon recess led to its withdrawal, however, and the Mayor ruled a similar new motion out of order. At the same session of the Council, a motion for the reinstatement of Miss Dyke was defeated.

On the 19th, the Council received an application for reinstatement from Miss Bullick herself, and also, a letter from Michael Kenny complaining about the way Miss Bullick had handled the case of his child. Both were forwarded to the Board of Control and then referred to the Medical Officer of Health with a request for a report on the latter. Dr. Jackson replied on 1 February that he had "read and carefully considered" the letter but he repudiated Mr. Kenny's charges:

> Without questioning the exactness of Mr. Kenny's statements, I yet am loath to think that, having in mind the tenets of their profession, any nurse could have exhibited quite the degree of harshness and indifference which may be inferred from this letter.[13]

Although there is no evidence to support the opinion, there was a rumour that "the last will and testament" of Charles Millar, an eccentric millionaire who had died in

Toronto in 1926, might have affected the case of the Kenny baby. Millar, who left an estate of close to a million dollars, had bequeathed the residue of his fortune to the mother who in the 10 years following his death had given birth in Toronto to the greatest number of children as shown under the Vital Statistics Act. According to a confidant of Millar, he believed that uncontrolled childbearing was the cause of much poverty and human misery, and he hoped, by turning the spotlight on unbridled childbearing, to make a laughing stock of Toronto and shame the Provincial Government into passing legislation to enforce birth control. The decade saw no great increase in the number of births in Toronto, however, despite the prospect of monetary award, but there were several women who had taken up the challenge, among them Mrs. Michael Kenny. The supposition of underlying rumour was that the public health nurses, aware of the fact and pestered by repeated unreasonable demands from the Kennys, may have been less zealous than usual in following through the case, especially when sensible and practical advice had been rejected.

The Millar will, which included several other equally bizarre bequests, was widely ridiculed and eventually tested in the courts on the grounds that "the stork derby clause" encouraged immorality. Finally, in 1937, Mr. Justice Middleton settled the matter by allowing the will to stand, and the legacy was divided among four women, each of whom had borne nine children during the 10 years following Millar's death. Mrs. Kenny, claimed that she had borne 10 children and should have received the entire $660,000. Her claim was disallowed, however, because several of her infants were either unregistered or stillborn. Nevertheless, to avoid further litigation, the winners voted that she be paid $12,500.

No action was taken on Miss Bullick's application, but at the first meeting of the Board of Control in the new year, the Mayor submitted a memorandum from the Legal Department of the City advising that Judge O'Connell had decided that she was entitled to compensation of $412.50 plus costs. The Judge had reasoned that, as a public health nurse Miss Bullick had had to have special training in addition to that of an ordinary professional nurse and, as positions for public health nurses were "by no means numerous in any municipality", vacancies did not occur frequently. Since her dismissal on 20 July 1932, despite "every reasonable effort", Miss Bullick had not succeeded in obtaining a similar post or any other for which she was trained except part-time nursing at the infants' home where she had worked since November at a salary of $58 a month. Further, she should have had at least three months' notice, and, as her annual salary had been $1650, and she had earned nothing during the three months following her dismissal, she was entitled to receive, "in lieu of compensation for wrongful dismissal", the equivalent of three months' salary plus $284.40 for costs.[14] Faced with this challenge, the Board of Control instructed the City Solicitor to consult the Corporation Counsel.

The Counsel, after studying the judgment, advised appeal to a higher court, because the Judge's decision had made it clear that existing City Statutes and By-laws relating to employment might have wide application. The Board of Control accepted his advice and ordered that an appeal be taken. At the same time, the Medical Officer of Health was instructed to obtain a copy of the Judgment and report his reactions. In his response, 3 January 1933, Dr. Jackson expressed profound disagreement with the Judge's opinion that factors of which he had been unaware might have altered his decision to dismiss or even to demote Miss Bullick. Despite his rejection of Mr. Kenny's charges, he still felt that "under the circumstances", the action he had taken was justified.

Meanwhile, the Mayor had called a special meeting of the City Council to report the recommendation of the Board of Control that an appeal be taken from the Judgment of Judge O'Connell. A subsequent meeting of the Council rejected the recommendation, however, and on 27 January, the Board of Control reversed its decision and ordered that the City Auditor be authorized to pay Miss Bullick the full amount stipulated by the Judge, $696.90.

Throughout the month of January, while the Board of Control and the City Council dithered over the question of the dismissal of the two nurses, including two motions for reinstatement, their supporters in the community had not given up. A further protest from the Local Council of Women, received by the Board on the 18 January, was filed without acknowledgement, and on 1 February, Mrs. A.L. Hynes, President of the Council, accompanied by a large deputation, presented in person 'various memoranda' (described by the press as a long memorandum) on the subject. In short, they believed that Dr. Jackson owed citizens some explanation. The Mayor replied, as he had done previously, that the question was "purely departmental in character" and should be dealt with by the responsible Head, the Medical Officer of Health. The women were thoroughly aroused, however, and, as in the autumn, *The Toronto Daily Star* took up their cause editorially as well as in reports of conversations with indignant individuals. There were charges that, if justice were not done by re-instating the nurses, citizens would no longer have any confidence in the Department of Public Health. The City Council should, therefore, *not* be deterred from doing its duty toward the two women, even if such action were to involve the resignation and dismissal of the Medical Officer of Health.[15]

The Globe, on the other hand, took the position that, in their zeal for re-instatement of the nurses, the Local Council of Women should beware of establishing a precedent that "could be but a step to further control of civic business by some Tammany organization, the sort of racketeering that has bedevilled administration in several United States cities".[16] There were, also, two women who wrote to the Mayor and City Council in support of the action of the Medical Officer of Health. Neither cited the stand taken by *The Globe*, but one of them complained that it hurt her sense of right to be represented by the horde of women of "befuddled imaginations" who had bombarded the City Council.[17] The other, whose letter was a copy of one she had written to *The Toronto Daily Star*, found the "prattle about JUSTICE nauseating". She had nothing personally against either Miss Dyke or Miss Bullick. They were simply part of a system that the public had accepted because they believed all that the late Dr. Hastings told them. She then trailed off in rhetoric about an unrelated case that had raised her ire.[18]

Not all Councillors were satisfied that justice had been done, and, on 7 February a motion similar to one that had been tabled by the Board of Control on 17 January 1933, was put before a meeting of the Council:

Whereas Miss Bullick was awarded damages in her action against the Corporation of the City of Toronto for wrongful dismissal and whereas there appears to have been grave injustice done to Miss Bullick and Miss Dyke by their dismissal from the Department of Public Health, be it resolved that it is the opinion of this Council that Dr. Jackson should re-instate the nurses at the earliest possible moment.

Rejection of the motion by a vote of 17 nays to 11 yeas brought the case to a close.

Still the newspapers could not forego comment. A *Star* editorial, "Council Votes to Continue Injustice", stated that Mayor Stewart had told the Council that the controversy was undermining the Health Department. "We believe", wrote the Editor, "that nothing could undermine it more than the knowledge which this vote conveys . . . namely that there is no remedy for injustice; that a wrong once done must stay done . . . . A great body of the electorate has lost faith in Toronto's health officer. That is unfortunate for the city and unfortunate for Dr. Jackson".[19] *The Globe* again took the opposite view: "In declining to order the re-instatement of two nurses dismissed by the Medical Officer of Health, the Toronto City Council took the only course justified by a clear view of civic administration . . . the question was whether the Council has the right to dictate – not whether the Health Officer had acted properly".[20]

Dr. Jackson having been determined to be rid of the two nurses, if the vote for their re-instatement had been unanimous, the Council would have had no alternative but to dismiss Dr. Jackson, since power of appointment to the staff of the Department of Public Health was vested in him as Medical Officer of Health. As it was, he remained in office until his death on 14 August 1951 and was succeeded by his deputy, Dr. L.A. Pequegnat, who is remembered as a much more competent Medical Officer of Health.

As a footnote to this episode, it is of interest that in all records of the Division of Public Health Nursing references to Miss Dyke's withdrawal mention a resignation, not a dismissal. Even though they felt that she had handled Miss Bullick's defence badly, the nurses recognized that she had laid a sound foundation for the development of public health nursing in Toronto.

The fact remained that she had joined the ranks of the unemployed. She was 49 years old and may well have looked forward to ten or fifteen more years in the post that had tested her mettle and refined her skills. What should she do? Where could she turn? She faced not only loss of a job and a regular income, she was humiliated, defeated and alone, remote even from the remaining members of her family. Moreover, the threat of deepening economic depression cast its shadow on the future.

HUNDREDS IN THRONG TO HONOR MISS DYKE

Many Messages of Tribute Read at Royal York Reception Last Night

HAILED AS PIONEER

Miss Dyke Asks Citizens to Support Public Health Nursing

The high esteem in which Miss Eunice Dyke is held by the citizens of Toronto, their gratitude for the part she played in not only conserving the health of the community but also in adding to its vitality, was evidenced last night at a reception tendered the former head of the nursing division of the civic department of public health in the Royal York hotel.

By the many hundreds who thronged the banquet hall, men and women from all walks of life, Miss Dyke was hailed as a pioneer in the field of public health nursing and as one of the first to give proper recognition to the value of preventive medicine. She was eulogized as a "faithful public servant" and tribute was paid to her 21 years spent in assisting to build up the health department to a point where it attained world-wide recognition.

From far and wide Miss Dyke received messages of congratulations on the honor. They were read to the meeting by Mrs. J. P. Hynes, president of the local council of women and chairman of the committee in charge of arrangements for the reception. Lady Falconer, chairman for the evening, presented Miss Dyke with a purse of money as a token of appreciation by Toronto's citizens for her work.

Played Vital Part

"For 21 years Miss Dyke played a vital part in all the outstanding movements in the interests of public health in Toronto," was the tribute of Dr. Minerva Reid, on behalf of the medical women in the city. Dr. Reid told of Miss Dyke's untiring efforts when Toronto was in the grips of two serious influenza epidemics.

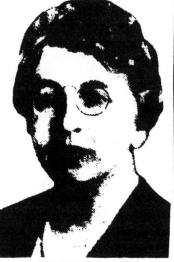

MISS EUNICE DYKE
Former supervisor of public health nursing in Toronto, Miss Eunice Dyke who was honored at a mass meeting held in the concert hall of the Royal York hotel last evening, when tribute was paid by women of Toronto to her work. There was a large number of prominent citizens at the meeting, who expressed appreciation of Miss Dyke's work. Junior League members acted as ushers.

—Photo by Ashley and Crippen

The Toronto Daily Star, *6 May 1933*

Chapter Nine

A Rockefeller Fellowship

Despite her summary dismissal, Miss Dyke's pioneering work was by no means unrecognized by her fellow citizens. On 5 May 1933, a public reception in her honour was held in the Royal York Hotel with Lady Falconer presiding. Miss Dyke was given a beautiful bouquet of flowers and a substantial cheque as "tangible expression of the spirit of the gathering". Dr. H.J. Cody, Sir Robert Falconer's successor as President of the University of Toronto, spoke about "the happy blending between official and voluntary work" that Miss Dyke had brought to the City of Toronto, and, on behalf of the medical profession, Dr. Minerva Reid praised her courage and foresight in giving "proper recognition to the values of preventive medicine". This kind of tribute was heart-warming, and Miss Dyke was deeply moved. In her reply, she included her nurses: "I realize that ... you are speaking through me to the public health nurses. If I may speak for them, may I ask for assurance of your constant support for them."[1]

Nevertheless, these were dark days. She wanted to "forgive and forget", but she was wracked by a sense of injustice. "What is the difference between charity and justice," she asked the minister of her church. He tried to be helpful, but the bitterness persisted. She must get away from the public eye even though 'the public eye' was, on the whole, indifferent to her dilemma. Then came a ray of light in a letter from the International Health Division of the Rockefeller Foundation addressed in care of Jean Gunn of the Toronto General Hospital, one of her most loyal friends. The letter asked whether Miss Dyke would be able to accept a fellowship for a year's study in the United States, beginning in the autumn, the writer none other than Mary Beard, whom she had known when she was studying in Boston in 1915-16. Now an associate director of the International Health Division of the Foundation, Miss Beard wrote that it would be a privilege to offer Miss Dyke a nursing fellowship. Rockefeller fellows from Europe who had been sent to Toronto owed much to field experience under her direction.

Miss Dyke accepted with alacrity. The prospect of a fellowship gave her "a great personal happiness", and she believed it would bring pleasure to many "as a means of minimizing the effects of recent civic episodes". Buoyantly she set off for Pointe au Baril on Georgian Bay.

Life in the Georgian Bay country was primitive and physically demanding. To fetch milk and mail, she had to row for two hours and a half every evening, and in early June the mosquitoes were vicious and inescapable. Gradually, however, the insects subsided, and she wrote to her doctor, "I am eating and sleeping as usual. The only change is the development of muscles from constant rowing and tramping on the rocks." The bold beauty of the rocks and trees enchanted her, recalling the painting of Tom Thomson and the Group of Seven.[2] Miss Dyke also enjoyed quiet hours of fishing among the shoals. But thinking was torment. "It is desperately lonely," she wrote to a friend who had sent her *The Autobiography of Lincoln Steffins.* "Reading and all civilized activities are difficult." She continued to feel, however, that getting away had been the wisest step for all concerned. "When the time comes for decisive action, I shall be ready," she declared.

But the time seemed never to come. Weeks dragged on with no further word of the fellowship, and then Miss Beard wrote that, because of "a great shortage of investment funds", all travel grants had been delayed. Not even the Rockefeller Foundation was immune from the devastating effects of economic depression. Miss Dyke undertook to nurse a local woman who had had a stroke, and it helped her to know that she had not lost the skills of bedside nursing which she had laid aside now more than 20 years ago.

Finally, in the last week of August, word came that a fellowship would be available. First, however, she must fill in and return various application forms and, when these had been reviewed, she would be informed of the Foundation's decision.[3] She decided to remain at Pointe au Baril until she could "speak freely of the immediate future", but she felt obliged to explain to her patient's son that he might have to make other arrangements for the continuing care of his mother. It was then, Miss Dyke explained, that she learned that he was local correspondent of the Toronto newspaper that had supported the nursing cause.[4] It would seem that the stroke her patient had suffered must have affected the woman's speech. Otherwise, with mothers' proclivity for talking about their sons, she would surely have told Miss Dyke about the son's occupation. In any case, the word was out. The 30 August 1933 edition of *The Toronto Daily Star* carried an account of the award with Miss Dyke's photograph under the headline: NURSE FIRED BY CITY WINS ROCKEFELLER SCHOLARSHIP.

The paper had been in touch with Miss Gunn who explained that from time to time the Foundation gave these fellowships to individuals in various countries. During her nursing career in Toronto, Miss Dyke had come into contact with many Rockefeller students who came to the city to pursue their studies, and the guidance she had provided for them, as well as her own record of achievement, were reasons for the award, one of very few that had been given to Canadians.

Apprehensive lest "premature notices of the fellowship" might have violated some regulation of the Foundation, Miss Dyke returned to Toronto. She saw only members of "the immediate family" and a few friends, but, even to them, she was unable to confess her embarrassment. Eventually an official letter dated at New York, 7 September, confirmed the award of a six-month fellowship to begin about the first of October, and she was able to enjoy congratulatory messages from friends and former colleagues, one of whom spoke of "vindication from the authority in your profession". To Mary Beard she wrote, "I confess to pleasure in these developments but am trying to keep the vindication spirit subordinate to other more important things," and she ended her letter with a lighthearted, "au revoir."

Preparation for a prolonged absence occupied the rest of the month. There were friendly farewells, details to be cleared with United States Immigration and shopping to be done. She bought a new winter coat and some 'other essentials'. There were letters to be written about the date of her arrival in New York and where she would live in the great city. She suggested 8 October as her beginning date, and it was agreed that she would live at International House, a residence for international students at 500 Riverside Drive, close to the campus of Columbia University, where she would meet interesting people from all parts of the world.

Life in New York City.

With introductions from Mary Beard, Miss Dyke lost no time in getting in touch with centres of public health nursing in New York. At the same time she was looking into possibilities of study at Teachers' College of Columbia University and discovered a study group on "Problems and Field Studies in Nursing Education". This interested her because she wanted to explore the relationship of private philanthropy to the development of public health and welfare agencies. "I find myself considering all activities that come under my observation in light of their negative or positive influence on the development of official activities," she wrote. If she could organize her reading and thinking along that line, she felt it would heighten the value of conferences with individuals of diverse experience. Withal, it was strange to be considering administrative questions without reference to an existing organization. The loss of her job of 21 years had left her without a mooring. However, her immediate concern was that, with a stipend to cover only living costs, she could not afford the tuition fee of $40.00, and it seemed to her a large sum for the Foundation to pay as an extra on her behalf. Miss Beard thought the fee not exorbitant and assured her that, if she felt the course would add to the value of her fellowship experience, the Foundation would be glad to pay it.

Association with the study group proved to be as rewarding as Miss Dyke had foreseen. Each member of the class was responsible for a group conference on a particular topic, and most of the time was spent in research. Happily, the sessions, held on Friday afternoons, fitted into her schedule. Fridays and Saturdays were not acceptable to field agencies as observation periods, and the mornings of those days gave time for the reading she needed to do. The other days she usually spent in observation visits to health centres, hospitals and social agencies, her only difficulty being how to select from among the many 'possible contacts' those that would be most valuable.

Eunice Dyke had an inquiring mind, and her interests ranged widely. She enjoyed "triumphing over a statistics primer" that had given her trouble, and she was intrigued by a report about district health centres that opened up questions of the roles and relationships of hospitals, field agencies and universities in nursing education. Already her experiences were throwing light on Canadian problems. She wanted to study plans for maternity nursing care in the Visiting Nurse Service of the Henry Street Settlement; in particular, its educational methods and how the Service cooperated with hospitals and with the municipal department of health. A visit to the Guggenheim dental clinic had given her some insight into "the health situation" in New York, and she hoped for further conversations with the responsible nurse. So it went, one contact led to another. Best of all however, was "the opportunity to do the kind of thinking that was not possible under normal conditions". Sometimes she had to explain that she spoke for herself only and not for the Rockefeller Foundation. "New York does not seem to mind challenging visitors," she wrote on 1 February 1934 to a friend in Canada, and added, "You see I am not out of line with Einstein's appeal to non-conformity". Nevertheless, she confessed that sometimes the result of her "long mental travels" reminded her of the mountain that brought forth a mouse.

One of those 'mental travels' was the planning of a system of records for a unified public health nursing service that she hoped might also be applicable to social case work agencies. If so, it would make possible a community rather than an agency basis for research. As time slipped by, this project became more and more absorbing. To test its validity, she got in touch with a wide circle of professional people—nurses, social workers and physicians and began to think of it in relation to her newly awakened interest in state medicine.[5]

As she travelled about New York, visiting one agency

after another, the subways and elevators that at first she had found intimidating lost their terrors. She began to see beauty that she had refused to believe existed. Mary Beard laughed at her when she called New York a town. "It is a continent," declared Miss Beard, but for Miss Dyke the 'town spirit' was a reality. She felt it especially when, visiting the city hall, she looked down from the roof toward the lower end of the city. Inevitably, she recalled conditions as she knew them in Toronto. "Even the most desolate appearing homes, if you can call them homes, do not seem to have lost more of the kindliness of home life than is lost in Toronto homes under adverse material conditions." She admired the sense of concerned citizenship that seemed so alive in the great metropolis. She found it in the New York newspapers, which, although "crowded with international news", did "not omit criticism of the U.S.", and she was baffled as she remembered the attitude of Toronto papers that were critical of all things American.

All the while she was warmed by the hospitality of people she was meeting in agencies that she visited, several of whom invited her to their homes. "One of the delightful surprises that New York has held for me is that many of the apartments have open fireplaces, and guests knit while they talk," she wrote. On such occasions talk must have turned to the political and economic ferment of the time that so closely touched the concerns of her new friends in New York. Four years after the crash of Black Thursday, 24 October 1929, the nightmare lingered. There were millions out of work (New York City alone had had a million and a half unemployed), and the industrial index had plummeted. Then had come the election of 1932 and the ringing words of Franklin Roosevelt's inaugural address of March 1933," ... the only thing we have to fear is fear itself, nameless, unreasoning, unjustified terror." Quickly the New Deal had been launched with anti-depression measures affecting banking, industry, agriculture and relief for the unemployed. They followed one after another: the Civilian Conservation Corps (CCC) supplied work for 250,000 jobless men of 18 to 25 in reforestation, road construction, and prevention of soil erosion. Part of their meagre wages went to their dependents to ease the harshest edge of poverty. An appropriation of 500 millions was made for emergency relief. The Agricultural

160

Adjustment Administration (AAA) was created to restore farmers' purchasing power.

There were other revolutionary measures, all bolstered by F.D.R.'s inimitable 'fireside chats'. In June, Congress had passed the National Industrial Recovery Act, umbrella for a series of programs under a National Recovery Administration (NRA). They were to formalize fair trade, establish competition codes and guarantee labor's right to organize and bargain collectively, while the Public Works Administration (PWA) was to increase the number of available jobs and stimulate business activity. Still business slumped in mid-1933, and shortly after Miss Dyke arrived in New York, an emergency unemployment relief program was introduced under a new set of initials (CWA, for Civil Works Administration). Its aim was to put people to work, not to support idleness with a dole, and no less than four million jobless individuals found jobs in federal, state and local 'make-work' projects. All this had come none too soon for the winter of 1933-34 was bitterly cold and plagued by drought, floods and hurricanes. By mid-January 20 million people were dependent upon federal relief for the essentials of living, and CWA needed more money. Glimmers of hope filtered through the apathy of despair as the recovery measures were implemented, testing the skill and integrity of administrators.[6]

Daily Miss Dyke was meeting individuals who were coping with the colossal problems of making new ideas work at the local level in New York City. To a friend at home she wrote, "New York is a wonderful place for visiting health and social workers just now, particularly as I have entree to much active thinking about changing milieux." Almost all those she met were involved directly or indirectly, but her reports highlight two women in particular: Katherine Tucker, General Director of the National Organization for Public Health Nursing, and Jane Hoey, a social worker, Secretary of the Health Division of the New York Welfare Council.

Miss Tucker, who was in close touch with complex problems of administering national relief, described some of her experiences. Miss Dyke was especially interested in a project in New York State that hired 117 previously jobless nurses to give bedside nursing care and health advice to

161

more than 60,000 needy families in upstate towns and cities. When things were well under control, along came inexperienced relief workers, who insisted that patients be removed from their homes to hospitals to save money, so they thought, and the nurses had to prove beyond doubt that home care cost less.[7] For Eunice Dyke it was an exercise that confirmed her long-time advocacy of home nursing care as both efficient and economical.

At the time, Miss Tucker was busy with follow-up of a recent Child Health Conference that had been convened in Washington by Frances Perkins, the Secretary of Labor. Despite efforts to reduce the effects of underfeeding of children during the winter of 1932-33, there had been a continuing increase in infant mortality, and the Conference was convened to consider how to find out the extent of the problem and what to do about it.[8] The subject interested Miss Dyke, but she decided not to get involved lest she spread her energies too thinly. Moreover, she had become intrigued with Miss Hoey's work as a public health administrator in New York City. They had some good talks about it, and Miss Hoey invited her to attend a consultation of representatives of member agencies of the Health Administration and Education Section of the Welfare Council to be held on the 31 January 1934.

It was an impressive group of people representing the City Departments of Hospitals and Health, New York Academy of Medicine, United Hospital Fund, New York Tuberculosis and Health Association and the Welfare Council of New York City. They had been called together to draw up a plan for placing health workers so as to provide services in health centres according to the distribution of patients in need of treatment in particular areas of the city. The project was one of several sponsored by Mayor La Guardia and the Commissioner of Hospitals and Health whose concern was to take advantage of CWA funds to place as many jobless health workers as possible as soon as possible. Miss Dyke felt privileged to see and hear the group at work, and her interest was further aroused by the fact of La Guardia's sponsorship. Fiorello La Guardia, elected Mayor of New York City in December 1933, was, next to Roosevelt, probably the most dramatic political figure of the time. Although a Republican and so briefly in office at that time, he was already taking advantage of resources available through the New Deal for the relief of the jobless and needy in his city. A member of the Italian community of New York, all his life he had resented the Irish faction of Tammany Hall which had become the centre of graft and corruption in city politics, and, having ousted them from power, he was on the way to becoming a legend – 'the Little Flower', three times re-elected to office as Mayor of New York and in 1946, appointed Director of UNRRA, (United Nations Relief and Rehabilitation Agency). According to his biographer, Arthur Mann, helping others gave La Guardia a sense of power and achievement.[9] His humanitarian spirit captured Miss Dyke's imagination, and to be associated ever so slightly with a project with which he was identified gave her deep satisfaction. He was one of the Americans whose exploits she liked to talk about on her return to Canada.[10]

Little wonder her days in New York were so filled that, in her own words, she had time to see "disgracefully little of the things visitors were supposed to enjoy in New York" – museums, art galleries, plays, music and window-shopping on Fifth Avenue. She did enjoy some diversions, however. Early after she arrived she wrote to her family in Toronto that Mary Beard had invited her to go see *Ah Wilderness*, a play by Eugene O'Neill. It had opened at the Guild Theatre on 2 October and on the following day had been favourably reviewed by Brookes Atkinson in *The New York Times*. Miss Beard thought that they would be "interested in the same points" and looked forward to them seeing the play together. Miss Dyke was embarrassed not to have known the play but was moved by the pathos of O'Neill's portrayal of an ordinary American family rent by petty despair and tortured adolescence in a small town in Connecticut in 1906.

As for music, among her papers there is a program of a harp recital at International House on a Sunday afternoon but, although there must have been similar concerts, one finds no mention of them. On the whole she liked living at International House, but in a letter home she described "a hilarious Hallowe'en Party" that she was "too old to enjoy". She had been a passenger in a stunt put on by 'the British group' about a sightseeing bus in New York. She thought the organizer had muddled through with too little planning, and

163

the megaphone man was vulgar rather than funny. Eunice hoped to learn that he was not British.

Among her fellow residents was one, Sara McCord, who was setting out on a holiday journey via the Panama Canal to California. Miss Dyke gave her a copy of *Magnificent Obsession* by Lloyd C. Douglas. That and *The Autobiography of Lincoln Steffens* seem to have been the only non-professional books that engaged her attention during this period. The latter she finally read in New York and returned to the friend who had sent it to her at Pointe au Baril. Apart from professional reading, which plainly she took seriously, and an occasional romantic novel, she appears not to have been "a reader" – an opinion confirmed by one of her nieces.

On one of her first Sundays in New York she went to morning service at Riverside Church. Sitting in the gallery she admired the architecture and the blending of colour between the building and the congregation that filled the nave. The gallery, she reckoned, held as many worshippers as the entire Park Road Baptist Church in Toronto, of which she was a member. About the sermon of the eminent Dr. Emerson Fosdick, she was less enthusiastic though not unimpressed. He had begun with the Scripture, "thou vain man, know ye not that faith without works is barren", and, without minimizing the problems, he talked about reconstruction of the social order. "He is certainly death on the profit system," she wrote, and while she agreed with him that the truth of Christianity must be proved in action, not in abstract theorizing, she decided that one of his sermons in a day would be "quite enough".

On a Saturday shortly after her arrival in New York, having already met six other Johns Hopkins alumnae, she went to "a Johns Hopkins tea", but there is no further mention of association with fellow graduates of the renowned School of Nursing. During that first month, she also did some shopping, her largest purchase a tailored suit for which she had to pay more than she had planned. She thought it wiser to buy it rather than a dress because she could wear it under her topcoat through the late fall. "I have always felt more comfortable in a suit with a wash blouse than in a dress," she wrote to her family. Not knowing the city well, however, she found shopping time-consuming and often frustrating. Distances were great, and she did not know where to go for what she needed, such as a new crystal for her watch or even a hair cut. She had looked everywhere for Rowntree's plain York chocolate but finally gave up, concluding that New Yorkers were addicted to milk chocolate. These trivialities seem to have been what she thought would interest her family.

Early in December, invited by Annie Goodrich, Head of Yale University School of Nursing, she went to New Haven to attend a conference, and while there met several people to whom she later turned for advice about her case record project. Then, later in the month, Barbara Blackstock wrote that she and Dr. Cody were to be married on 27 December and would be in New York for a few days at the end of the year when they hoped they might see her. Impulsively Miss Dyke wrote to Mary Beard to ask whether, in view of the Codys' wide influence in Toronto, and their interest in education and public health nursing, it might be possible for them to visit her office. As always, Miss Beard responded cordially suggesting various officials whom they might meet, though she herself would be out of the city. Since the Codys were in New York for a very short time, encounters such as these, which Miss Dyke felt "might help matters in Toronto", were out of the question. She continued however, to count on the friendship and understanding support of Mrs. Cody.

Years of economic depression in the United States had brought a rise in sickness, especially among the new poor who could not afford to consult a doctor. Health centres under municipal auspices were overcrowded, while private physicians waited in vain for patients, and, without adequate preventive measures, the health of the nation was deteriorating. A study conducted by the Milbank Memorial Fund confirmed a growing conviction among health and social workers that the country must work toward a national health plan. As Miss Dyke became aware of these developments, the subject of health insurance interested her increasingly, and she began to think of her health and social care record system as a useful tool in implementing a comprehensive health plan. Feeling that she needed more time to consult key individuals in the health field in order to perfect her project, she was loathe to leave the stimulating environment of New York. Early in the new year, therefore,

165

she asked to have her fellowship suspended for the months of February and March, to be resumed in April. The two months then remaining she proposed to spend in Canada, "on British soil", observing relationships between public and private health and social agencies and consulting about possible uses for her record-keeping system. On enquiry, Miss Beard found that, with her approval, this plan would be acceptable to the Foundation, and Miss Dyke was enabled to remain longer in the U.S.A. and to visit New Haven again, this time for consultation about her project.

While in New Haven in December, Miss Dyke had met Dr. C.-E.A. Winslow Professor of Public Health at Yale University Medical School. He was renowned for his advocacy of public health as a community service dependent upon the cooperation of several disciplines,[11] and she thought that his opinion of her project would be invaluable. With Miss Beard's acquiescense, therefore, she sent him a wire on 8 March asking if he would be willing to challenge her idea for "a basic health and social care record". She told him also that she hoped Misses Goodrich and Fox whom she had met as a Red Cross nurse when she was in Paris in 1924, and Mrs. Winslow would join in challenging the scheme. Anne Rogers Winslow had been a fellow researcher with her husband before their marriage in 1907 and had continued to work closely with him. It occurred to Miss Dyke that, if this group thought her proposal practicable, Dr. Winslow might arrange to have it considered by a committee of the Institute of Human Relations, with which he was associated.

Dr. Winslow replied that he had signed up the group for a meeting at his home at three o'clock on Monday, 19 March, and then came a letter from Mrs. Winslow inviting her to spend Sunday and Monday nights in their home. They were having parties both evenings that they thought she would enjoy. Overwhelmed by this proffered hospitality, she accepted, saying that it would be "a very sun-making piece of the road", and she would even be prepared to have them think her community case record merely visionary. For Miss Dyke it was an unforgettable week-end, "one of the happiest of this surprising winter", even though the discussion of the case record study was inconclusive. After 15 minutes, one of the New Haven nurses remarked that the scheme contained no new ideas, and the others "did not consider it an orthodox case record form". Dr. Winslow, however, promised to consult some of the staff of The Institute of Human Relations and give his opinion later, but Miss Dyke's papers give no evidence of what that opinion may have been.

During the intervening week, she had attended some sessions of the Annual Conference of the Milbank Memorial Fund[12] and was particularly interested in 'a round-table' on national health planning chaired by Dr. Winslow. Discussion focussed on the scope of a plan for compulsory health insurance proposed by Dr. I.S. Falk of the Fund's research staff. He advocated benefits in service, rather than cash, for individuals and families in large groups, preferably on a state-wide basis. The plan allowed for free choice of a physician and adequate payment for all professional personnel involved in treatment and administration. Various means of finance were suggested – federal subsidy, state and local taxation or all of these, together with contributions from insured individuals and employers. Dr. Falk estimated that the cost would be little more than Americans were already paying in "hit and miss ways" in amounts that were beyond the resources of increasing numbers of citizens. The Conference commended the proposal and recommended that it be submitted for discussion to professional and lay groups, the latter to include employers and employees. There were guests present, however, who favoured wider scope. For instance, Mayor La Guardia would have preferred a national rather than a state-wide basis, and Harry Hopkins, Federal Relief Administrator, urged the Conference to be bolder. "You are not going to get health insurance if you expect people to do it voluntarily," he declared. "I am convinced that by one bold stroke we could carry the American people along not only for health insurance but also for unemployment insurance. I think it could be done in the next 18 months".[13] This was heady stuff, and Miss Dyke was gratified that her experience had led her into interests that were dominating the thinking of leaders in health and welfare in the U.S.A.

Miss Beard, meanwhile, had been expecting her to submit an itinerary so that the Foundation could make arrangements for her travel in Canada during the remaining period of her fellowship, but Miss Dyke kept putting the matter off. Anxiety about what she might find at home crowded her mind. Would anybody share her enthusiasms

167

and her concerns? Must she expect hostility, especially from doctors who remembered the long-drawn-out dispute in Toronto? Would there be a job for her? She could not bear the thought of being excluded from the health field. "My hope for the years ahead is to be closely in touch with patient care but with a perspective that will use any position I hold to bring about the general application of high standards of care of the sick as part of health promotion. In some inconspicuous position I may foster community planning. I am seeking such a position in Canada," she wrote to Miss Beard, adding that it was from that point of view that she had sought advice from Dr. Winslow and his associates about her ideas for case record-keeping on a community basis. As for her fellowship period in Canada, in her visits to hospitals, she felt she must avoid becoming absorbed in patient care and the use of ward and clinical facilities for the training of nurses. Rather she resolved to concentrate on community planning.

With these factors in mind she had written to consult Elizabeth Smellie, Chief Superintendent of the Victorian Order of Nurses for Canada, and Charlotte Whitton, Executive Secretary of the Canadian Council on Child and Family Welfare. Both these women, working from headquarters in Ottawa, were aware of current developments in health and welfare throughout the country. Miss Smellie was a long-time friend and nurse colleague whose judgment Miss Dyke respected. Miss Whitton she had never met, but the Council on Child and Family Welfare was an instrument that she thought might bridge the gap between voluntary organizations and government. In 1920, shortly after the creation of a division on child welfare under the direction of Dr. Helen MacMurchy in the Dominion Department of Pensions and National Health, the Deputy Minister, Dr. J.A. Amyot, called together in Ottawa representatives of all child welfare agencies, both public and private, to form a voluntary council or clearing house to work with the new departmental division. As a result of that meeting, the Canadian Council on Child Welfare was formed, its purpose "to correlate efforts in child welfare, compile information and develop educational activities". It was voted an annual government grant of $1,000, which, in 1921, was increased to $5,000. At first the Council had an honorary staff, but additional funds from private sources enabled it to open an office in 1926, and Charlotte Whitton, who had acted as honorary secretary, was appointed full-time executive secretary. Three years later, at the request of social agencies, family work was added, and it became the Canadian Council on Child and Family Welfare. Miss Whitton was a dynamic personality in the field of social service and, since 1922, had served as a delegate of Canada to the Committee on Social Questions of the League of Nations. To have caught her attention was for Miss Dyke a highly gratifying experience.

Both women replied at length, but of the two Miss Dyke thought that Miss Whitton had more readily grasped what she had in mind. Province by province, she had cited examples of cooperation between health and welfare agencies, both public and private, and named individuals whom Miss Dyke should consult. In Vancouver the City Relief Officer and the Provincial health authorities were giving $1,500. a month for medical care of dependent families in their homes, and through the Financial Federation, a health service had been built up for all agencies in the 'community chest'. As well, Dr. G.M. Weir, now Provincial Secretary, had "quite definite plans for public health and state medicine". For information about recent developments in social services in Alberta and Saskatchewan, Miss Whitton recommended articles in the journal, *Child and Family Welfare*. Winnipeg, she wrote was about to adopt a broad scheme of health services for dependent families, and Toronto was "very much torn as between public and private services". In fact, that question was so much to the fore in different parts of the country that a committee had been appointed to study the situation and try to draft a national statement that would give some direction. Meanwhile, Ottawa already had underway a project to provide medical care for relief recipients in their homes. Master mind of the plan was one of the leading surgeons in the city, and it was being worked out under the Public Welfare Board. Miss Whitton suggested that Miss Dyke spend sufficient time in Ottawa to meet the people close to the project, which she described as "a most complete experiment in certain phases of public medicine". Montreal came into the picture, too, with comment on the complex relationship between French and English agencies. All these developments she felt sure would interest Miss Dyke.

Also, she thought that both the Canadian Conference on Social Work with community planning high on the agenda of its meeting late in May, as well as the annual meeting of the Canadian Public Health Association in Montreal in June, would add grist to Miss Dyke's mill.[14] All in all, Miss Whitton had given her the kind of information she thought she needed.

Miss Smellie, on the other hand, wrote in general terms, her observations spiced with drollery. She knew of no unusual developments in nursing service, only much talk and little action, because no one had any money. She reminded Miss Dyke that Canada had no NRA or "correspondingly revolutionary alphabetical processes". Social work had made some advances because, in difficult times, the trained worker had proved a wise investment, but avalanches of work had prevented the keeping of adequate records. There were too many over-riding problems. Visits to Ottawa and the capital cities of the provinces would give her plenty of food for thought and better understanding of the difficulties of administration in a country so vast, with competing federal and provincial jurisdictions. The British North America Act had become 'a football', either the greatest obstacle or the best safeguard according to the point of view of whoever was writing or talking about social, or, indeed, other national issues. Nevertheless, Miss Smellie had no doubt that a strong national leadership along medical and social lines, if available in an advisory capacity, could benefit the country enormously. She also mentioned a recent Order-in-Council that, following Dr. Helen MacMurchy's retirement as Chief of the Division of Child Welfare in the Department of Health and National Pensions, had authorized transfer to the Canadian Council on Child and Family Welfare activities of the Division that belonged more properly to the sphere of a voluntary organization, an incident that Miss Whitton had omitted from her comment on cooperation between government and voluntary agencies.

In a later letter, Miss Smellie gave her the names and addresses of district superintendents and supervising nurses of the V.O.N. She also suggested key people, including nurses in charge of nursing services in city health departments, and advised writing to the Red Cross, whose work in the western provinces she thought would excite Miss

Dyke's interest. For instance, the Society had struggled to develop some good plans of cooperation with official agencies. Her most forthright advice, however, was in response to something Miss Dyke must have written about her dread of publicity.

> As to your being conspicuous, you may as well face it right now that newspaper reporters will be on the door step . . . to ask what are your impressions of the particular place, the people in it and the work they are doing. The West is like that. I think it arises from their genuine desire to give all guests an enthusiastic welcome so that when they go home they will have a very vivid recollection of kindness and hospitality without stint. (13 March 1934).

Advice was helpful, but it was time for action. Miss Dyke left New York on the first of April. She had decided to go directly to Vancouver, visit Victoria and travel eastward, visiting centres in each of the provinces of Western Canada. Having been granted a further suspension of her fellowship, from 14 to 27 May, she would spend the time 'at home' and go to Hamilton for the Conference on Social Work. From 1 to 10 June she would be in Ottawa and then finish the period of her fellowship in Montreal from the 11th to the 19th. She would have liked to have fitted in a visit to Nova Scotia, but Miss Beard cautioned against so much travel in so short a time. In any case, the fellowship did not allow for travel in two directions, and she wanted to be in Montreal when the Canadian Public Health Association would be meeting. If she could avoid Dr. Jackson, she would attend some of the sessions. Then she would go to Hamilton for the Conference on Social Work and finally, to Toronto, for the annual meeting of the Canadian Nurses Association. She dreaded a return to that "point of conflict" but knew that she must face it.

By 1934, doubtless as a result of the great depression, railways had already begun to deteriorate. From New York to Chicago Miss Dyke had a rough ride. "A pen is impossible on this road, and even a typewriter is erratic", she wrote. Nevertheless, only two days out of New York she had typed two letters to Miss Beard. Her mind was by no means at rest about the future. She hoped to avoid conversation with reporters and was apprehensive of misunderstandings with nurses and organizations that she might encounter.

Vol. XXX

MONTREAL

JANUARY 1934

No. 1

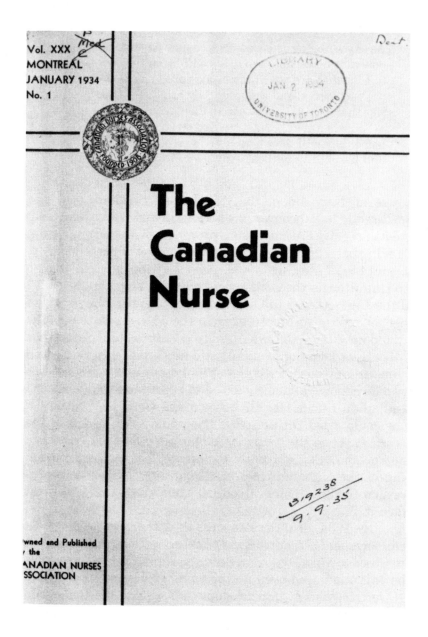

The Canadian Nurse

Owned and Published
by the
CANADIAN NURSES
ASSOCIATION

Chapter Ten

Return to Canada

When the immigration officers at Portal on the Canadian border accepted without comment her "letter of explanation" from the Rockefeller Foundation, Miss Dyke was 'at home' again, once more on what she called 'British soil'; her mind enlivened by her American experience. To Floyd Lyle of the Foundation's Fellowship and Travel Service, she wrote:

> The journey over the prairies and through the Rockies and Selkirks was a very beautiful one. The sun shone so brightly that we were compelled to wear snow glasses for the mountain section. (8 March 1934).

"Vancouver," she added, "was at its sunny best with flowers everywhere." She arrived there on Saturday, the 6 April, and booked in at the Hotel Vancouver. Then Miss G.M. Fairley, Director of Nurses in the Vancouver General Hospital, to whom she had written from New York, started her happily on her way.

Her first official conversation was in Victoria, with Dr. H.E. Young, Provincial Health Officer, who immediately afterward wrote to her, "We are living at the end of the line and do not have the pleasure of meeting many like yourself whom we would like to consult". Under separate cover he sent her copies of reports on public health work in the schools which they had talked about. Dr. Young was concerned about health care in camps for unemployed men for which he felt nurses could not be given responsibility. However, Miss Dyke thought the difficulties not insurmountable and later in her travels, she took up the argument by correspondence. The Provincial Director of Mental Hygiene in Saskatchewan had told her that he sought the best women available among the nurses to staff the male wards of provincial institutions. "He considers that male attendants alone are not equal to the task," she wrote. "Why couldn't the Department of Pensions and National Health find and appoint nurses who could assist with the administration of those camps?" There is no record of a reply from Dr. Young.

Miss Dyke was reminded of the early days with Dr. Hastings when she met several Vancouver physicians who were interested in community policy. Here, the Toronto situation was reversed. While Dr. Hastings had involved the nurses in community planning, it had been difficult to persuade the doctors to assume leadership. In Vancouver, on the other hand, the doctors were taking the initiative and were impatient with the indifference of the nurses. One doctor she described was reminiscent of the old family physician tradition in a new milieu. "He was agonizing over case records as everyone does who is trying to give direction to medical, nursing and allied services in the public health movement," she wrote. She gave him a copy of her community case record which she thought might steer him away from some of the difficulties he was having.

She was critical of social workers whose reactionary attitudes, she thought, belittled the capacity of qualified workers in their own profession by discouraging their appointment to positions in the civic services. Eager to air ideas, she tested her notion of social service as a function of hospital head nurses and internes, with social workers as special supervisors who would take over cases referred for intensive study, on Miss Beard. She thought a scheme like that might make doctors more 'teachable' and social workers less 'high hat'.

There was little time for sight-seeing or other diversions, but Miss Dyke spent an evening playing bridge with three nurse friends and "kept them up far too late". The high point of her visit, however, was a conversation with Dr. Hill of the University "to whom the nursing profession owed so much", now retired and living in West Vancouver. "We agreed," she wrote, "that the value of getting to principles is that they apply anywhere." She had come to the conclusion that there should be *more* organizing of the community and *less* of the professions.

Miss Dyke left Vancouver reluctantly and, travelling by Canadian National through the mountains, arrived in Edmonton on the 17 March. In the higher altitude of Alberta she had more energy than at the coast and later wrote of the enjoyable and enlightening time she spent in that province. Following an interview with the Deputy Medical Health Officer, Dr. M.R. Bow, she drove with Miss Brighty, Provincial Director of Nursing Services, to several smaller towns. They saw a mental hospital in Ponoka and municipal hospitals in Innisfail and Red Deer. In the latter town, they also visited a school for the mentally deficient and a health unit "that was paving the way for state health insurance". Insufficient time to enquire about curative work in the health unit left Miss Dyke groping for light on administrative and legislative aspects of health insurance that would necessitate cooperation from the nursing profession. Her confidence was restored and her imagination stirred, however, by a visit with a district nurse who was responsible for health care in a remote settlement where there was neither a hospital nor a doctor. The nurse was living in a log cabin built for her by neighbours, near and far, some of whom she and Miss Brighty enjoyed meeting. The contribution of their labour had helped to bind the community together, and the log cabin was "the centre of hospitality and culture for the neighbourhood".

Back in Edmonton, Miss Dyke found "evidence of retardation of nursing vision" which she feared might hinder the development of public health programs. The Medical Health Officer of the City was an energetic young man, but his work was made "unnecessarily difficult by the isolated thinking and experience of his otherwise splendid nurses". Under these circumstances, she decided to avoid meeting him. She did not want to talk with a health official about such problems until she had had a chance to discuss them with Miss Smellie. Miss Dyke was often unduly hard on her fellow nurses but always careful not to share her misgivings with outsiders.

After Alberta, she went on to Saskatchewan, where years of drought and plagues of grasshoppers had denuded the land and left near-starvation in their wake. Hundreds of farmers and unemployed city-dwellers were living on a meagre monthly relief cheque and an annual clothing allowance of $40 for a family of four.[1] No other province of Canada suffered so severely as Saskatchewan during the bitter years of the thirties. Miss Dyke had not realized the extent of misery and distress, and she was moved by the slogan, "Just one more crop!" which she heard everywhere. She was also aware of 'cross currents' caused, she thought, by the impending provincial election. In fact, they were stirrings of political radicalism of varied stripes, including principles of democratic socialism espoused by the recently organized Canadian Commonwealth Federation (CCF), one of whose advocates was a Baptist minister– none other than the Rev. T.C. Douglas who was a candidate in the election.[2] Social change was in the air.

In Saskatoon, Miss Dyke's first stopping place in the Province, arrangements had been made for her to meet Dr. W.C. Murray, President of the provincial university, an interview that at the time seemed to her pointless. Later, however, she felt that Dr. Murray had given her insight into "the Saskatchewan mind". The splendid new university buildings planned by a Montreal architect and built of stone from glacial drift, became for her a symbol of the resilient faith of the people and their hopes for the future.

Chiefly, of course, she was in touch with health personnel– nurses, doctors, provincial and municipal administrators of public health, all of whom were coping with health problems beyond their resources to meet. In both city and countryside there were diseases like trachoma that flourish under conditions of poverty. With a provincial public health nurse, she visited a trachoma treatment centre near Saskatoon that was typical of others throughout the province. The nurses devoted a large part of their time to ensuring that the proper treatment was continued at home and that the causes of infection, often a towel used in common, were removed. Yet the disease persisted among pre-school and school-age children as well as adults.[3]

In Regina, Dr. Middleton, the Deputy Minister of Health, was cordial and helpful, and Miss Dyke found much in common with Ruby N. Simpson, the Provincial Director of Nursing Services, who was President-elect of the Canadian Nurses' Association. On the other hand, however, the city medical officer of health was, in Miss Dyke's opinion, a weak administrator. The school health program had not been integrated with the work of the Department of Public Health, and Miss Simpson explained that the city lacked a qualified nurse who could develop a coordinated administration of the two services. In contrast, the nurse in charge of the Victorian Order was "able to think beyond her immediate task", and the work of the Welfare Council was progressing well under the direction of a social worker from the east. Miss Dyke was gratified, too, when she found that the training of student nurses in the Regina Central Hospital included two months in the psychiatric department. Although she was not sure why, visits to mental hospitals had been a major part of her program thus far, and judging from what she had seen in now three provinces, she decided that the training of nurses who were entrusted with mental patients was hopelessly inadequate. In her conversation with Dr. Murray, she told him that she would like to visit a mental hospital at meal times or when patients were being put to bed. Murray replied that each province would doubtless prefer that she make such a visit in another province. It so happened, however, that she spent her last night in Saskatchewan as a guest of the director of nursing in the mental hospital in Weyburn and was taken on an evening tour of the wards, an experience that whetted her concern.

"What is to be done about this matter?" she wrote to Miss Brighty, and writing to Miss Beard, she partially answered the question: "I realize that some way must be found for the nursing heads of these services to confer together without obstacles imposed by medical and political authorities". She was not sure which of these authorities she feared more, but was convinced that first steps toward a solution of the problem must be taken within the nursing profession itself. With the same zeal as years before she had struggled to achieve recognition of the role of public health nurses and adequate training for them, she was now ready to tackle similar issues relating to nursing services in mental hospitals.

From Regina to Weyburn she travelled by bus through one of the worst sandstorms of the season and, visiting in the environs of both cities, she got an inkling of the hardships of rural people. She visited a one-room school to which children trudged for miles across the flatlands, and she saw a broken-down hospital building that served as headquar-

177

ters for one of the province's public health nurses who brought hope and healing to people in the surrounding area. Her next stop was in Winnipeg, where a long conversation with Dr. F.W. Jackson, Deputy Minister of Health for Manitoba, "no relation whatever to the Toronto one", helped her to see through the maze of conflicting ideas in medical and nursing services in the western provinces. Depressed economic conditions had led to increasing confusion, even antagonism, between public and private services. There were health units served by municipal doctors and nurses, municipal hospitals, and in some municipalities, private physicians were paid out of public funds for the care of patients in their homes or in hospital. Nurses had varying roles, from private duty to public health work and were employed under various auspices – provincial or municipal governments or private organizations such as the Victorian Order. Dr. Jackson also confirmed an impression of resentment of the Victorian Order, which Miss Dyke had formed during her visits in the other three provinces where she had been told that the Order was invading public health functions of government nursing services.

The problem of the V.O.N. reminded her of similar tensions affecting the nursing services of the Henry Street Settlement in New York. The key to continuing growth and usefulness of that service had seemed to her to be the ability of the head of the nursing division of the New York City Health Department to weave non-official services into the fabric of the municipal services. In the case of the V.O.N., Miss Dyke thought solution of the problem would require larger numbers of statesmanlike nurses on the staffs of municipal agencies. She discussed the matter with Ethel Cryderman, a former staff nurse of the Toronto Department of Public Health who had felt repressed under Miss Dyke's leadership. Now in an executive post with the Victorian Order, Miss Cryderman was staying in the same hotel as Miss Dyke in Winnipeg, and they discussed the work of the Order. Miss Cryderman thought that, because the V.O.N. depended upon lay boards and dealt directly with the public, its nurses must be more outstanding than those who served the community through a municipal agency. With this point of view Miss Dyke did not agree, but, despite differences of opinion, or perhaps because of frank expression of them, she

178

enjoyed meeting Miss Cryderman again.

While in Winnipeg, she also had helpful exchange of experience with Ethel Dodds Parker, whom she had known as Chief Welfare Officer in the Division of Welfare of the Toronto Department of Public Health and later, as Head of the City's Welfare Department. At the request of the Winnipeg Council of Social Agencies, Mrs. Parker was making a survey of family services in Winnipeg for the Canadian Council on Child and Family Welfare. With these two former colleagues, Miss Dyke discussed the keeping of records of community care services for which public grants were made. She had been compiling data on "a case basis" in the cities she had visited and was delighted to have a chance to explain her plan for centralized records to knowledgeable individuals.

Her program in Manitoba was confined to Winnipeg because of the City's strategic position in the Province but had been imaginatively planned by Miss A.E. Wells, another former Toronto nurse, now on the staff of the provincial department of health. Interviews had been arranged with a variety of people whose work Miss Wells knew would interest her: the local medical officer of health; a statistician who was also director of child welfare; the nurse in charge of the city's school health services; the medical director of the Workmen's Compensation Board, who had ideas about "precedents for state health insurance"; a physician who was a member of the Economics Committee of the Canadian Medical Association; the medical superintendent of the psychiatric hospital, and the medical officers of two health units. She also talked with the Secretary of the United Farm Women, the Director of Women's Institutes and several other prominent women, among them Mrs. J.F. (Margaret) McWilliams, at that time the only woman on the City Council, whom she had known previously through a shared interest in child welfare. Miss Dyke was especially gratified, also, to meet three nurses who, as hospital superintendents, were responsive to her concerns.

Climax of the visit was a dinner party under the auspices of The Manitoba Association of Registered Nurses when, as guest speaker, Miss Dyke talked about her experiences as a Rockefeller Fellow in La Guardia's New York and in the provinces further west. The occasion gave her opportunity to introduce ideas that she wanted to foster: socialized medicine, nursing as a function of government and the importance of the study of civics which her encounter with the Winslows had highlighted. Writing to Miss Beard afterward, she remarked that, while her visit to Winnipeg might have seemed to have had no specific purpose, it had worked out naturally and acceptably. She had been especially happy to discover that Winnipeg nurses realized that there would be need of leadership from nurses, if socialized medicine in any form were to be introduced.

The visit had been a gratifying conclusion to her period in western Canada, and she left for Orillia feeling "torn between inclination to seek opportunities to help with the evolution of the public health field and an urge to seek opportunities to retreat from it".

Returning to the east, she looked forward to two weeks' respite in Orillia, a pleasant town 130 kilometres north of Toronto at the south end of Lake Couchiching, later famous as the prototype of Stephen Leacock's *Mariposa*. Having known the place since childhood, she would feel at home. She would clear up correspondence and reflect on her recent experiences. Perhaps, too, she might get some sense of what she might do next. It was endlessly depressing not to be able to answer queries about her plans for the future. The hostess of the Old Home Inn, where she would be staying, had promised her protection from newspaper reporters, and travelling from the west, she could reach Orillia without going first to Toronto, an ordeal that must be faced eventually.

From that haven she wrote to the Winslows about her study of public health services in the western provinces which she felt had given her an inkling of the Canadian approach to socialized medicine. She had found some agreement about the usefulness of a central record of services to individuals and families, including its effect on the public purse. Unfortunately, in most communities, files were so scattered that to bring them together would be a formidable undertaking. Nevertheless, she thought it would be worth while to try out her scheme if it be only as a control on purchase of the services of private physicians. Moreover, it might encourage the use of home nursing care as a part of socialized health services. Paradoxically, she added that it had been distressing to find her own ignorance shared by many of the nurses she met – perhaps a reflection of inadequacy she felt in the midst of the élite group in New Haven. In any case, she believed that the limited outlook of otherwise competent nurses was hampering "statesmanlike medical officers", an idea that she had already expressed in letters to Miss Beard. In closing she struck a lighter note as, with a touch of nostalgia, she recalled the Winslows' hospitality. She asked them to pat the dogs and take a glance for her at the lovely Connecticut Valley.

As days passed, she was diverted by the pleasure of renewing acquaintances in Orillia, where she had taken care of her Aunt Tilly. She played bridge with friends, one of them, a summer resident whom she had known as a member of the Toronto Board of Health who, because of her interest in civic affairs, was claimed as 'a real citizen' of Orillia. Another was a public health nurse, a student in a special course at the mental hospital in Whitby, who had been sent to Orillia for field work with the two community nurses. There was a good hospital in the town, and Miss Dyke glimpsed possibilities of new developments in public health work. Finding that the Reeve, who was acting mayor and a member of the hospital board, was interested in the idea, she suggested that Kathleen Russell be asked for help in securing a nurse with public health training as superintendent of the hospital and its training school. To Miss Beard she wrote, "This town and vicinity would be ideal for health unit purposes ... I believe that all the essentials are here ...." It occurred to her that, if she were to seek wage-earning work in Orillia, the problem of her immediate future might be solved. As an established citizen of the town, she would be able to foster the growth of community health work.

In better spirits, she set out for Hamilton where she was welcomed by the director of the City's recently organized division of public health nursing who engaged her in discussion of the problems of the new job. This was the kind of challenge she had longed for, and drawing on both her Toronto experience and insights she had gained in New York, she felt secure in advising the nurse about how to cultivate good working relationships within the Department of Public Health and in the community as well. She herself had made enquiries about the Hamilton post while still in New York and, except for proximity to Toronto, would have welcomed it. However, that was the past, and now the future – her future – was uppermost in her mind, and feeling confident that her advice had been useful, she gave her imagination wing. If only she had an adequate income or could capitalize on her experience, she might carve out a rewarding place for herself in Canada as a research consultant in nursing. For instance, nursing as a function of government was a subject that ought to be explored. Canada employed nurses in the army, in prisons, in general and mental hospitals and also in provincial and municipal departments of health. In addition, private duty and Victorian Order nurses were sometimes brought into public service. In-depth study of these diverse roles might yield information that would convince the nursing profession of the significance of its relationship with government and advance the day when education authorities would assume responsibility for nursing education.

The Conference on Social Work, which she had attended, left her discouraged about the prospect of partnership among professions concerned with community welfare. She had thought that the Canadian Council on Child and Family Welfare might provide a channel of cooperation but had come away feeling that social workers wanted to control every situation, while the other professions did woefully little community thinking. Perhaps social workers should be trained as general practitioners in case work and community organization with other professions providing technicians and specialists in their own fields. She would have preferred, however, that there be equal partnership in defining and developing respective professional functions. Thinking of the record system she had struggled with, she concluded that she had been making a more or less conscious effort to influence staff education toward integration of services to meet the needs of individuals and families. To that end, however, her efforts seemed thus far to have been of little use. Even so, she was reluctant to give up the goal of partnership.

The Council on Child and Family Welfare in Ottawa was, nevertheless, still very much on her mind. She had been told about the recent withdrawal of a nurse from the staff, leaving a vacancy that she might be eligible to fill. Although the work of the Council was oriented to social work and seemed to her to be dominated by social workers, she had learned that, ever since 1926, the staff had included a nurse as secretary of its division on maternity and child hygiene. In those eight years, however, five nurses had held the post, and one after another had either resigned or been asked to do so. *If* she were offered the job, what should she do? She was meeting friends whom she thought she could consult but found them reluctant to give advice. However, she had got an impression that the source of difficulty lay, not in the combination of a social worker and a nurse, but in the personality of the Executive Secretary. Despite Miss Whitton's admittedly outstanding ability, she failed to sustain the confidence of associates. Nevertheless, Ethel Johns, who represented the Canadian Nurses' Association at the Conference in Hamilton, believed that a nurse was needed on the Council staff, a strong individual who could find ways for the nursing profession to participate in the Council's program. Mrs. Cody, who had herself recently resigned from the Board as a result of incidents that had destroyed her trust in Miss Whitton, advised her to accept a temporary appointment if opportunity offered, and Jean Gunn suggested that she "go off the deep end".

On the way to Ottawa, travelling in the same railway car, she and Miss Whitton had their first person-to-person meeting, and a few days later Miss Dyke wrote a letter to Miss Beard, telling the whole story of the previous days, including also the encounter on the train: "Miss Whitton is small, dark-haired and inexhaustible physically and mentally. She is a protestant with an understanding of the Roman Catholic elements in the country which is the result of a mixed milieu in childhood. She worked her way through Queen's University . . ., helped to educate younger members of her family, is a member of the University Senate and was a member of the committee which sought the president in the old country . . . She is intimately acquainted with the professional and governmental personnel of Canada and has represented us at Geneva."

There was more of Miss Whitton's life history, including reference to the Council but no mention of the staff vacancy that interested Miss Dyke. Miss Whitton did, however, explain the Council's current relation to the Government, which (as Miss Smellie had written) had recently been extended by Order-in-Council. In December 1933, the Department of Pensions and National Health, instead of replacing Dr. Helen MacMurchy on her retirement as Director of its Division of Child Welfare, had turned over to the Council services of the Division that seemed to be more properly activities of a voluntary body. This action had raised a storm of protest from people who thought it a retrograde step to transfer a government service to a private agency. Miss Whitton however, had ignored this opposition. She believed the arrangement would give the Dominion Council of Health and the Canadian Medical Association time to decide what they want in the way of a federal health department. The Government grant to the Council had been increased to provide for an anticipated increase in service but only by an amount sufficient to sustain the enlarged responsibility. Moreover, there was nothing in the Council program that could not be omitted in case of a change in public policy. Currently the Council, in cooperation with provincial authorities, was carrying on an educational service, making available to interested individuals and organizations publications dealing with maternity and child hygiene. The provinces liked this arrangement, probably because all publications bore the imprint of the authority that distributed them. Under these circumstances, Miss Dyke concluded that the country owed Miss Whitton "a vote of thanks".

Obviously, Miss Dyke had been captivated by Miss Whitton's ability and her strength of mind. At the same time, however, she recalled that her friends had described the woman as a politician who condemned, condoned or admired people according to their attitude toward her own achievements. Yet a job on the Council staff would be a bonanza, and to Miss Beard, she wrote, "I am unhappy about my feeling of caution". In Ottawa, conversation with Miss Smellie and other V.O.N. staff members confirmed her hunch that she was being considered for the job, but they offered no advice. Gertrude Bennett, Superintendent of the Ottawa Civic Hospital, who was a member of the Council executive and a close friend of Miss Whitton, was equivocal. She intimated that, while the appointment might be desirable, it could create difficulties for both Miss Dyke and the Council. There was a brief meeting with Miss Whitton, who asked for her help in finding a strong nurse to fill the post, and she suggested that Florence Emory, then President of the C.N.A., put forward a name.

At various social functions, Miss Dyke met old friends, both nurses and social workers, and in talk with the Medical Officer of Health, she learned that he was interested in medical education. He had just returned from a visit to Kingston and had high hopes that Queen's University medical school would decide to use Ottawa's clinical facilities. Miss Dyke was enthusiastic about such a possibility as an enrichment of the city's public health program which, she felt, here as elsewhere, was hampered by doctors treating nurses as subordinates rather than associates *and* by the nurses accepting that relationship.

Her own immediate dilemma dominated her thinking, however, and she decided to cut short her visit to Ottawa and go on to Montreal where she hoped she might get better perspective on the problem. In that city, the Annual Meeting of the Canadian Public Health Association held her attention for a few days, but it took second place to her dismay at the cleavage between the English minority and the French majority – the tragedy of Canada of which she seems not to have been aware previously. She wrote:

> Educational systems are distinct; health services under official auspices are one; the health services under private auspices are distinct. The nursing departments of the two universities are distinct in organization, and there do not appear to be any effective personal contacts.

Under these circumstances she could see little hope of building an efficient public health service, but she could not leave the matter there, and she added: "If the barriers of race and language could be dissolved by accepting the differences as an educational asset instead of a problem, we might make a small experiment for the League of Nations!"

Nothing, however, could take her mind off the Council vacancy. She went to see Dr. A. Grant Fleming, now Professor of Preventive Medicine in the McGill University Faculty of Medicine. He had been associated with the Council as first Chairman of the Division on Maternity and Child Hygiene, and Miss Dyke, of course, had known him earlier as Deputy Medical Officer of Health in the Toronto Department of Public Health.[4] Ostensibly, her purpose was to find out what he thought about the role of nurses in a system of socialized medicine. Actually, she wanted to consult him about a possible future for her as successor to the five nurses who had filled the Council post now vacant. Dr. Fleming, like the others with whom she had discussed the matter, emphasized the difficulties in personal relationships that were likely to occur.

While in Montreal, she heard from Miss Whitton that Miss Emory had refused to give any advice, giving as her reason that already five nurses had been unable to handle the situation. Nevertheless, Miss Johns, with whom Miss Dyke discussed Miss Emory's reply, was convinced that, in spite of difficulties, a nurse who would have confidence in the Council must be found, and she advised Miss Dyke not to close the door. Then, on 20 June, the day after her Rockefeller fellowship came to an end, Miss Whitton came to Montreal to interview her and, after a long conference, they agreed that the interests of both Miss Dyke and the Council would be best served if an appointment were made on a temporary basis, if at all. Miss Whitton asked her to return to Toronto by way of Ottawa for an interview with the appointment committee, but, wracked with uncertainty, she refused, explaining that she wanted very much to visit a niece in Cornwall on the way home.

Three days later, she arrived in Toronto to find a tracer telegram which was followed shortly by a special delivery letter offering her the position for six or nine months as might be decided by the Board and asking for an immediate reply. Without more ado, she telephoned her acceptance.

All that had happened on Saturday. Then on Monday, came a second special delivery letter from Miss Whitton reporting that some influential members of the Board thought Miss Dyke might not be in sympathy with the educational service of the Division for which she would be responsible and might try to eliminate it from within. The letter merely stated, however, that, while grants that maintained the Division on Maternity and Child Hygiene were designated for educational services, other types of service might also be developed in future. She was told also that questions had been raised about 'personality difficulties' for both herself and Miss Whitton. She replied giving assurances of her loyalty to the Council and to the Executive Secretary throughout the period of her appointment and afterward. She added, however, that she would like to be sure that life insurance companies that helped to finance the Division would not oppose any form of socialized medicine that might be approved by federal and provincial departments of health and/or the Canadian Medical Association.

Charlotte Whitton, by now plainly eager to complete negotiations, answered by return post giving 'reasonable assurances' about the attitude of the life insurance companies and later wired to say that the Canadian Medical Association received an annual grant similar to the one made to the Division. She suggested, however, that, while still in Toronto, Miss Dyke get in touch with Hugh H. Wolfenden, who was retained for research work by the Canadian Life Insurance Officers' Association. Miss Whitton also asked her to see Dr. J.T. Phair, Director of the Child Hygiene Division of the Ontario Board of Health, who had recently resigned after seven years as Chairman of the Health Committee of the Council. Mr. Wolfenden was out of the city, but she had a talk with Dr. Phair who suggested that, with her outlook and experience, she should be able to create an entirely different situation from the one that had defeated her predecessors. Undoubtedly Dr. Phair would have been one of the influential people who were being consulted about the appointment. Dr. G.P. Jackson was another, and Miss Whitton had assured her that he raised no objections. Here then were prospective supporters she could count on, one of them her former enemy, yet he had not stood in her way at the crucial moment of a Council decision. Surely this was a favourable omen.

Meanwhile Miss Dyke's suitability for the post had been high on the agenda of the selection committee in Ottawa which comprised two nurses, Miss Bennett of the Civic Hospital and Miss Smellie from the V.O.N.; two recently appointed medical consultants of the Division, J.F. Puddicombe, Obstetrician, and L.F. MacHaffy, Pediatrician; The President of the Council, Dr. R.E. Wodehouse, who was Deputy Minister of Pensions and National Health, and Miss Whitton as Executive Secretary. Other possible candidates were quickly disposed of, and attention focussed on

Miss Dyke whose appointment was urged by the two nurses. The doctors, on the other hand, feared "kickback from the blow-up in Toronto", and Dr. Wodehouse agreed to consult Toronto physicians, Drs. Jackson, McCullough, Chief Health Inspector, Department of Health of Ontario, and Phair, by telephone. None of these three anticipated serious backlash, while Drs. Jackson and McCullough went so far as to say that they would like to see Miss Dyke in the post. Dr. Phair, however, though convinced of her ability and the soundness of her professional qualifications, thought difficulties might occur in working arrangements, especially in relation to the Executive Secretary of the Council. Describing the discussion in a letter to Dr. J.H.T. Falk, Executive Director of the Vancouver Council of Social Agencies, Miss Whitton wrote: "The point of view seemed to develop very generally that Miss Dyke could bring tremendous experience, undoubted standing and a real contribution to this Division far beyond that of any other nurse in Canada, but that she offered grave difficulties in working with other people which would flare up when a person like myself had to work with her". Plainly Charlotte Whitton underestimated the difficulty she herself presented in working with other people, especially some one of equally strong mind. Esther Beith, who knew both women well, thought the appointment should be given serious consideration but with the safeguard of a temporary clause, a suggestion to which Miss Dyke had already agreed. The committee accepted that proposal, recommending a time-span of from six to nine months.[5]

Final decision remained with Miss Whitton, but she wanted wider opinion and, dramatizing the situation, she wrote: "I feel a bit like Ramsay MacDonald when Britain entered the war ... There are such strong currents both ways that I cannot possibly take the responsibility again myself and have let the matter be decided by a majority opinion of the Board on the basis of a circular letter I sent them". Replies to the circular fully endorsed the committee's recommendation, and on 29 June, Miss Whitton posted a letter of appointment that Dr. Wodehouse as President of the Council had endorsed.

The letter, which reached Miss Dyke on the following day, informed her of her engagement to join the staff of the Council as Secretary of the Division on Maternity and Child

Hygiene from 10 July to 31 December 1934, and explained the duties, staff relationships and the lines of accountability involved:

> You will take the responsibility of heading up this Division, of continuing, consolidating and improving its present programme, and of suggesting any expansion or improvement in that programme. You will have associated with you ... Doctors MacHaffy and Puddicombe as medical staff, and Mme Chasse in the French-speaking health services. Your work will tie in to the General Council through the Chairman and Vice-Chairman as members of the Board of Governors and through me as executive officer.
>
> ... the Division will operate with considerable autonomy as to its technical programme, but considerations of policy ... will continue to rest finally with the Board of Governors, with whom all questions of finance and of the Division's expenditures will rest.
>
> In December, the Division executive and the Board of Governors will review with you, this preliminary six months' work with the Division, and on the basis of that experience, and your own inclination, will determine the question of permanent appointment to the Division Secretaryship. We confidently anticipate a most satisfactory development of our work from your leadership in its organization at this time.
>
> The salary will be at the rate of $2,000 per annum.

The press took little notice of the appointment, and Miss Dyke concluded that she was no longer news, but the August edition of *The Canadian Nurse* gave it an entire page under the title, "An Interesting Appointment":

> The Canadian Council on Child and Family Welfare has announced the appointment, for a limited period, of Miss Eunice Dyke as secretary of its division on maternal and child hygiene. This division is one of eight which unite in an effort to advance the standards of home and national life by seeking to create throughout the Dominion of Canada an informed public opinion on problems in the field of social welfare. The Council endeavours to assist in the promotion of standards and services which are based on scientific principles and which have proved effective in practical experience.
>
> Miss Dyke brings to her new work years of experience in

relating the contribution of the nursing profession and private philanthropy to the responsibility of the official agencies.

There followed a summary of her achievements as Superintendent of Public Health Nurses in the Toronto Department of Public Health, with references, also, to her observation of public health activities in Europe in 1924 and her recent study and travel in the United States and Canada under the auspices of the Rockefeller Foundation. A final tribute completed the article:

> She is one of a growing group of pioneers who seek to relate nursing to the services of other professional and non-professional workers, on a community basis. There is probably no other nurse in Canada who possesses so broad a background in civics ... or as broad a knowledge of the principles of public health administration. The Council is to be congratulated on obtaining her services.

Early in July Eunice Dyke moved to Ottawa eager for this fresh challenge.

Chapter Eleven

Six Months Trial

As she opened her roll top desk at Council House in Cooper Street on July 10, Miss Dyke pondered, "Is it an auspicious beginning or isn't it?" In any case, it was a fresh start. She was undertaking an educational position, its emphasis none other than her long-time interest in preventive medicine and the health of the community. The program of the Division on Maternity and Child Hygiene was based on the premise that health education and the formation of good health habits could overcome preventible or remediable illnesses and defects caused by carelessness, indifference and malnutrition and thus forestall many premature deaths. The purpose of the Division was not, therefore, to engage in research but to disseminate and apply the facts of good health already known.[1] True, she would be working within a form of organization totally different from the Toronto Department of Public Health, but she believed in the aims of the Division and of the Council as a whole. Moreover, she was confident that, drawing on her long experience in public health and welfare work, she could help to advance those aims. To be or not to be a new career, the next six months would tell. This was no time to ruminate, so she set to work.

On her desk was a memorandum of unfinished business appended to a review of the work of the Division since its inception. It was a paper that Miss Whitton had prepared for distribution to members and to provincial health officials to describe Council services provided through the Division over the previous five years. Monthly letters on pre- and post-natal care and the health needs of the pre-school child had been edited and distributed on request to expectant and new mothers through provincial health departments and

Eunice Dyke as secretary of its division on maternal and child hygiene. This division is one of eight which unite in an effort to advance the standards of home

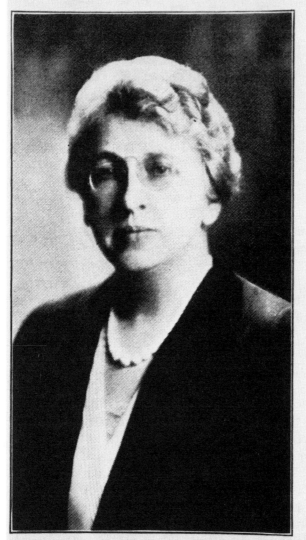

MISS EUNICE DYKE

and national life by seeking to create throughout the Dominion of Canada an

the Toron
nurse from
Nursing.
returned t
visiting nu
Public Hea
with that
Public Hea
one of its
system kno
she prefers

With th
ing efforts
ment of th
secured a
association
Boston, at
community
need for
existing s
She was t
preparatio
for public
is one of
who seek t
of other pi
workers, c

Miss D
tunities
activities i
pleted a
travel in t
under the
Foundatio
will doubt
for the r

The Canadian Nurse *records her new position*

the national office. This type of service had been initiated in 1926 by Dr. A. Grant Fleming, then Chairman of the Division, to provide medical advice to expectant mothers according to a pattern that had been developed by the Montreal Association on Child Welfare. There was also a diet-folder service, a project taken over from the Canadian Public Health Association, to explain rules of diet for children from infancy to school-age. 'Special publications', – folders, posters and charts– had been produced from time to time on recommendation of Division members. News stories and articles on health questions had been contributed to a selected list of periodicals. Staff members had spoken about Division concerns at conferences or during field visits, and radio talks and exhibitions of health literature had also spread the word. Presumably, most, if not all of these, were activities that would be continued in future.

What of unfinished business? Five items were listed: Preparation of a short and simpler edition of the pre-school letters to be translated and published in French, once the acceptability of the English version had been demonstrated; Initial planning of the number, frequency and the content of a school-age letter series that had been approved in December 1933; Publication of three charts bringing up to date the Council's charts on maternal mortality and infant mortality by cities and infant mortality by causes; News stories for publicity about the Council to go out on an average of one every three weeks, if possible. Routine matters, Miss Dyke thought, not matters of policy. Right now, however, she must set about preparing background material she had promised to send to Ethel Johns, Editor of *The Canadian Nurse*, for the article about her appointment to the Council staff. Also piled high in her office were publications of the Council Division for which she was now responsible. To these had been added a flood of literature from Dr. MacMurchy's bureau in the Department of Pensions and National Health. Some of the material might be discarded but most of it must be organized for accessibility. *And* a meeting of the Executive Committee of the Division had been scheduled for July 18. That should give her a better 'feel' for the job.[2]

The executive committee met infrequently to continue discussion of questions that had emerged in meetings of the entire Division, and detailed planning was left to a sub-executive consisting of the chairman, vice-chairman and staff of the Division. Members resident in Ottawa were also included to make possible quick convening of a quorum. The meeting on the 18th had been called to review decisions taken at a full meeting of the Division held on 14 June 1934, when members had been informed about what had happened since the Governing Body accepted transfer of services from the Division of Child Welfare in the Department of Pensions and National Health. Of all eight Divisions of the Council, the one on Maternity and Child Hygiene had been most affected by the transfer, but, except for the new section staffed by Drs. Puddicombe and MacHaffy, who were to provide medical information, the program of the Division, although slightly amplified, was not to be altered. Its function had been and would continue to be the production and distribution of literature and the conduct of other projects in the field of maternal and child hygiene. It was to these 'other projects' that Miss Dyke thought she might look for greater scope. The transfer did, however, make one change in the structure of the Division. The Department of Health had requested that a technical sub-committee be appointed, its membership to consist of a liaison officer from the Department, the secretary of the Division, the obstetrician, the pediatrician, the secretary of the French-speaking service and the Executive Director of the Council. This committee was to meet each month to consider matters of reference, including new projects or publications, and report its findings to the sub-executive committee.

Looking further into the Minutes of 14 June meeting, Miss Dyke noted that, in order to alert the public to the persistent problem of maternal mortality, the Council was arranging to have a health official from Britain tour the country. This decision, which was to involve her more closely than she realized at that moment, interested her especially. She was aware of the urgency of the problem as a result of her participation in efforts to grapple with it in Toronto.

Her attention was also caught by a two-pronged statement that had been added to the terms of the transfer of services and later confirmed by both the Department of Health and the Governing Body of the Council:

While the transfer of work is primarily concerned with the

Division on Maternal and Child Hygiene, it is understood that the whole development is to have the personal supervision of the Executive Director of the Council ...

The second part of the statement was in capital letters:

Notwithstanding any details of this memorandum, it is understood that ... the administration of all business of the Division and final disposition of all services of the Division shall rest with its own Executive and full Division ... under the chairmanship of the presiding officer of the Division.[3]

What was this telling her about the job she was undertaking and the degree of responsibility entrusted to her?

In the next few days she disposed of immediate tasks, including correspondence with various provincial officials about the availability of publications they had requested, and on the fourteenth, she wrote a memorandum to Miss Whitton about the disposition of literature within the office: duplicates and other valueless materials should be eliminated; pamphlets, pictures, texts of radio talks, newspaper releases, teaching projects and other materials worth retaining should be added to the library under appropriate classifications. Concise and definite, though imperious, her recommendations proved acceptable as did a request made through Miss Whitton's secretary that, for a time at least, all correspondence for the Division go to her desk. She wanted in particular, to see letters answered by the physicians, Drs. Puddicombe and MacHaffy, which would keep her informed about medical aspects of the Division's programs in which she had special interest. Also, pursuing her interest in the cost of medical care, she asked for and received from Dr. Fleming a copy of The Report of the Committee on Economics of the Canadian Medical Association.

When the Executive met on the 18th, she took up her role as recorder. Miss Whitton had introduced her as having been appointed Secretary of the Division for the period, 10 July to 31 December, but as she later explained, she withheld comment because of the length of the agenda. Had there been time, she would have said that a temporary appointment would permit the Council to review its policy and programs at a critical time, and the secretary to consider her qualifications for the post, thus avoiding the complications likely to arise from an agreement of indefinite time. Also, as the meeting progressed, she stated that she had not had a chance to consult the Executive Director but she hoped that, except for the most urgent matters, the items of the agenda might be discussed as opportunities rather than commitments. Miss Whitton intervened to say that the interests of the Division and of the Council would require an intensive, continuous campaign similar to the work of the previous five years. It was a directive that ruled out a suggestion from Dr. Young, Medical Health Officer of British Columbia, undoubtedly initiated by Miss Dyke, that a study of nursing services in Canada should be undertaken. Miss Dyke insisted, however, that she would like to consult the Director about the feasibility of a pamphlet on public health nursing.

More urgent matters claimed the attention of the Committee: concerns that would determine the design and content of Division program during Miss Dyke's agreed term of office. Keeping in mind questions raised at the recent meeting of the Division, the executive must decide about priorities for revising existing publications and preparing needed new ones. It was agreed, however, that a publication was not always the best way to introduce a subject. For instance, in response to anxiety about the effect of economic depression on the health of the nation, it was decided that, instead of a pamphlet on the subject, Miss Whitton, Miss Bradford (the executive assistant) and Miss Dyke should assemble data on the effect of the depression on morbidity and mortality as a basis for deciding whether to direct attention to the subject in Council propaganda for the extension of health services. The preparation of a pamphlet on poliomyelitis, urged because of recurrent epidemics, was also rejected because it would require epidemiological analysis beyond the scope of a voluntary agency. Miss Dyke pressed for immediate consideration of pamphlets on two other subjects: "Sources of material on health education for schools" and "Sex education in child welfare programs".[4]

Discussion ranged widely, and several meetings of the sub-executive committee were needed to continue the planning process until a program had been drafted for the remainder of the year. A decision was taken to undertake a study of how provincial authorities distributed the Council's health publications, including channels for local distribution.

In the end, it was also agreed to ask the Council to consider the preparation of three new publications: a pamphlet on sources of teaching material for child health centres; a series of letters about the mental and physical health of school children, and a pamphlet on principles and techniques of public health nursing. In this last suggestion Miss Dyke had triumphed. The final report stressed "two guide lines" for the Division's planning. First, because "health is one of many related aspects of life", the Division on Maternal and Child Hygiene must rely on the combined insights of all divisions of the Council in selecting and developing its activities. Secondly, consultation with representative officials of provincial departments of health would facilitate the discovery of acceptable sources of scientific knowledge and experience, a fact that might well be kept in mind in planning the tour of the British official, whose contribution to such discussion would be invaluable.

This was a formidable program for Miss Dyke's brief term of office. She was reminded of the story of the father who gave his sons bundles of faggots to be broken. Baffled at first, they found that the answer was to break them one at a time. This she must do. But scarcely had she broken a single 'faggot' when she allowed Miss Whitton to commit her to travelling through the western provinces with the visiting British official: this in addition to responsibility for correspondence with provincial and local agencies to arrange details of the itinerary! Annoyed at herself, she felt she had been outwitted. The prospect of a prolonged absence from Ottawa seemed like a nail in the coffin of her hopes. She suggested several "representative nurses" who would be satisfactory 'couriers', but Miss Whitton had made up her mind. Miss Dyke later wrote to Mary Beard, "As early as August, I realized that it would be impossible for me to influence the policies of my Division or even details within existing policies ...."

Despite low spirits, however, Miss Dyke was gratified by the account of the assignment in *The Canadian Nurse* which announced that "A Distinguished Visitor", Dame Janet Campbell, DBE, LLD, M.D., M.S. (Lon), who had recently retired as senior medical officer for maternity and child welfare in the British Ministry of Health and chief woman medical officer to the Board of Education of Great Britain, would be coming to Canada in October. "Accompanied by Eunice Dyke, R.N., secretary of the division on Maternal and Child Hygiene of the Canadian Council on Child and Family Welfare, Dame Janet will visit all the larger cities of Canada as part of an educational campaign to arouse greater interest in maternal welfare." The tour, the article explained, was being arranged under the auspices of the Canadian Council on Child and Family Welfare and various cooperating national, provincial and local services in the fields of health and welfare.[6]

Miss Whitton had written to Dame Janet on 11 August, outlining an itinerary and telling her that Eunice Dyke, a Registered Nurse who would accompany her on most of the trip, was preparing for enclosure a memorandum of some of Canada's problems relevant to the subject. Dame Janet's travel in Canada would begin from Quebec, where she would arrive on Friday, 12 October. On Sunday, she would go on to Ottawa and spend three days there before going west to Winnipeg, Regina, Saskatoon, Edmonton, Vancouver and Victoria. Returning east, she would visit Toronto, Montreal, Saint John and Halifax, from where she would sail on 28 November. In a postscript, Miss Whitton added that Miss Dyke's memo was not ready and, in any case, was unnecessary as she was enclosing several pamphlets. Miss Dyke finished the memorandum, however, and mailed it to Dame Janet. At the same time, she sent a copy to Miss Whitton, who returned it, having written in the margin that she found it very good but would have appreciated seeing it before it went to Dame Janet. Furthermore, she thought the Division's own report, "Maternal and Child Health Provisions in Canada and her Provinces", would have been more useful for a stranger coming to Canada than such a lengthy narrative. Miss Dyke did not reply but, later in the month, she wrote another long letter to Dame Janet with information about the cities to be visited, and the engagements that had been made for her.[7]

These time-consuming tasks, together with correspondence to arrange Dame Janet's program, diverted Miss Dyke's attention from the regular work of the Division. Nevertheless, she fitted in a speaking engagement in Saint

John early in September, initiated consultation with officers of the Dominion Bureau of Statistics about revision of the charts of infant and maternal mortality rates and wrote a letter for the Department of Immigration and Colonization to distribute to recent immigrants. Whether or not she assumed this letter would be translated into other languages is unclear but the text read:

> Sept. 14, 1934. A letter to immigrants from the Canadian Council on Child and Family Welfare.
> Ottawa is far away from your home, but we are interested in you and hope that you have found pleasant neighbours. We enclose a stamped envelope for you to tell us if you need advice at any time.
> Perhaps you may wish to ask a public health nurse near your home to visit you or may wish us to send you some of the publications in the list enclosed.
> Sincerely yours,
> Eunice Dyke, Registered Nurse.[8]

She also drafted the questions for the enquiry about distribution of Council publications on maternity and child hygiene. The survey she had in mind was highly detailed, inviting opinions about the form and content of publications, asking what, if any, duplication there was with material produced by the province itself, and how local distribution was carried out. There were questions, also, about the effectiveness of methods of advertising Council materials by its own staff as well as by provincial departments of health and local health authorities. While Miss Dyke was away from Ottawa, several provinces wrote to protest about the amount of work required to answer the enquiry, and Miss Whitton, obliged to apologize for the elaborate approach to the task, was not amused.

She had already been provoked by a memo Miss Dyke had written just before Dame Janet and she left Ottawa. A brief conference on the previous day had led Miss Dyke to think that a plan of propaganda for her Division to be submitted to the Dominion Council of Health would be drafted in her absence, and her memo outlined a series of arguments against this possibility. For the executive director and her assistant to initiate such an important project without the participation of the Division secretary would violate a principle of Council organization. She believed, moreover, that the prestige of the Council would be enhanced if a carefully matured plan were worked out in cooperation with interested national women's organizations, a process that would take time.[9] Miss Whitton, however, preferred to make policy decisions on her own.

Travel with Dame Janet was a refreshing contrast to the prickly relationships of everyday life at Council House, and Miss Dyke had the added satisfaction of renewing acquaintances with provincial officials whom she had met in the spring. She mistrusted Miss Whitton's motives in promoting the visit, however, and in contrast, found Dame Janet to be "a genuine person and an experienced public health administrator whose contacts had undoubted constructive value but not in the way that Miss Whitton intended ...." Moreover, Miss Dyke began to think that others shared her views about Miss Whitton's administration, and she even went so far as to claim that, in some centres, in order to avoid "a complete flop", she had to explain to health officials that their reception of the guest could be without prejudice to their opinions of the Council's national policies. Although, except on one occasion, she was not present when Dame Janet talked formally with provincial and local health personnel, she felt certain that Council affairs were freely discussed. She came to the conclusion that Dame Janet looked forward to conversation with Miss Whitton and would be able to help in shaping "a statesman-like policy". Not surprisingly then, the fact that the only occasion Miss Whitton arranged for an exchange of thinking with Dame Janet was "a two-hour luncheon interview" in Toronto was, in Miss Dyke's eyes, not only a discourtesy but also a lost opportunity. Nor was Miss Whitton's response to her own reporting of the journey any more reassuring. "She has not sought any information from me since my return," she wrote to Mary Beard, and added, "... there is so much help I could have given her which would have accomplished more for the Council and its funds than platform and newspaper publicity."

What seemed to Miss Dyke the ultimate in betrayal confronted her, however, on her return to Ottawa on 17 November. During her absence, the date of the Division meeting when her period of work would be reviewed had been set as 30 November, and an agenda endorsed by the Technical Sub-committee on the thirteenth, had been mailed to members on the fifteenth. Chief among the agenda items was the annual report "to be given by the Executive Director in view of the change in secretaryship in April...", and there was also to be "a special report by Miss Dyke". With the announcement of the meeting there were several enclosures, one of which was the same list of 'unfinished business' that she had been given in July. This time, however, beside each item was a precise suggestion for completing it, even to the names of the people who might be asked to undertake the task, either individually or as members of small working groups. It was the kind of direction that, had it been proposed five months earlier, would have expedited her approach to the secretaryship of the Division.

Further, to Miss Dyke's dismay, she learned that, at Miss Whitton's suggestion, her report would be studied by a committee of reference not later than 23 November, then forwarded to the Executive Secretary (she expected to be out of the city) by special delivery on the morning of the twenty-fifth so that she might return it with comment. The Technical Sub-Committee would then meet for further study of the report, which, with suggestions for discussion, Miss Dyke would present at the Division meeting on the thirtieth. After "these preliminary considerations", the report would be mailed to members of the Board of Governors of the Council on 1 December "for consideration before and at" their meeting in Toronto on the fourth.[10]

Angry and frustrated, Miss Dyke decided that she must not submit to this arbitrary planning and she found at least one ally in Dr. Fenton Argue, Vice-Chairman of the Division and Chairman of the sub-executive, who, although he had been present at the meeting of the technical committee when Miss Whitton's proposal was accepted, agreed that the action should not have been taken in the absence of the secretary of the Division. After further consultation, therefore, the proposed agenda was withdrawn, and Miss Dyke made only a brief report which she described in a letter to Mary Beard:

It expressed confidence in the future of the Division but indicated the future which I considered worthy of confidence. To the uninformed, it would mean nothing but to the informed would carry a message ... It anticipated further reports to the Executive Director and a responsible committee. It announced my withdrawal.

There was no doubt in her mind. She had come to the end of her association with the Canadian Council on Child and Family Welfare. "I anticipated difficulties but nothing so extreme," she wrote and added, "For financial and other more worthy reasons, I would have considered remaining but it would have meant serving Miss Whitton's personal interests and not those of the public. The thing was impossible."

The Governing Body, at its meeting on 4 December, authorized the appointment of a committee to study the role and relationships of the Secretary of the Division on Maternal and Child Hygiene. The Committee was to include representatives of the Canadian Medical, Dental and Nurses associations with the addition of several people who were not identified with the Council. It would work under the direction of Esther Beith, Secretary of the Child Welfare Association of Montreal. Miss Beith, who had earlier been on Miss Dyke's staff in Toronto, had been outspoken in the meeting of the Division Council about the changing nature of public welfare and the need to understand the relationship of social work and public health nursing in meeting community needs. Moreover, she believed that the Council on Child and Family Welfare provided common meeting-ground for the two professions to achieve fruitful cooperation.

Writing to Miss Beard, Miss Dyke commended this decision which she believed might pave the way for constructive changes. That the Council was facing a crisis there was no doubt but, despite misgivings about Miss Whitton's administration, there was general agreement that, were she to leave at that moment, the Council would die. Even so, Miss Dyke could not forego a last word:

> I am hoping that Miss Whitton will be big enough to avoid strategies, in which she is a master, to secure control of the Study Committee.

Miss Whitton was not the only threat to the Committee's work that Miss Dyke anticipated. She feared that representatives of the Canadian Medical Association and other opposing forces, which she refrained from naming, might be tempted "to destroy utterly a thing which might become a helpful ally of the national and provincial health services." Economic conditions were steadily worsening, and naturally her own situation was uppermost in her mind. Once again, she felt she had been caught in a situation where personal and professional ethics had been difficult to determine and she saw herself still bound up with the Council. There might be "stimulated misunderstandings", and if there were, she was not sure that she would be able to deal with them "without adding to the great difficulty of preserving the Council for an unknown but useful future".

With a heavy heart she returned 'home' to Toronto.

Chapter Twelve

Further Ventures

Coping with life in the 1930's

I believe Miss Dyke lived in the present and the future.
Ben Holmes

The journey back to Toronto was a retreat from hope. The events of 1932 rankled in Miss Dyke's mind, and the Ottawa venture had been another humiliation. She decided not to stop in Cornwall; it would have been unbearable to face her niece, Catherine Barrick, who lived there. Now she would be a failure to family and friends. At least, however, she had a place she could call home, "a genteel rooming house" at 644 Spadina Avenue, as she knew that her landlady, Miss Barwick, would have a room for her. She had moved there from the apartment in St. Thomas Street where her father and her brother Gordon had spent their last years with her. Miss Dyke continued to live in that house or in similar lodgings in other parts of the city until 1944, when she rented a small apartment at 40 Hazelton Avenue. At different times, in the following years, she made a home there for each of two grandnephews whose mother had died. The building was a 'walk-up', and she lived on the third floor. Nevertheless, undaunted by two long flights of stairs, she stayed in the same place for twelve years. A friend who knew her at the time has no recollection of the furnishings. She remembers only 'Miss Dyke', an imposing figure grappling with questions of the day, especially the plight of the elderly in a changing society.

The 'thirties were devastating years in Toronto.

204

Already before Miss Dyke left the city in the fall of 1933, there were growing numbers of men and women out of work. The public health nursing staff had been reduced, and there was a general ban on the employment of married women in professional work, and if a woman married, her job was in jeopardy. It mattered not that she might be highly competent in a post that required wisdom and experience. One such was Miss Dyke's former colleague, Ethel Dodds, since 1921, Chief Welfare Officer in the Department of Public Health, who had married Cameron Parker in 1923. Thousands in more desperate straits were unemployed, unable to find jobs. Destitute men from other parts of the country invaded the city and swelled the queues at soup kitchens in search of a free meal. Church halls and empty buildings were converted into dormitories to provide night lodgings. Relief costs soared. Many a breadwinner who had never asked for help of any kind had no choice but to apply for assistance. Yet, while Toronto had more than 100,000 relief recipients, it was said to have more than 10 millionaires.[1] Nevertheless, prices were low and, if one had even a little money, it was possible to manage.

Miss Dyke was one of those who had only a little, but, in the words of a friend, "she made do". According to her nephew, John Fox, who looked after her finances in the last years of her life, money meant very little to her. By standards of the time, she had had a good salary in the Department of Public Health ($3,150 in 1930) but she had not saved much. Her sister Winnifred thought her extravagant, or so said Winnifred's daughter, Mrs. Catherine Barrick. There had been a small legacy from her father's estate that had benefitted all his children, and her brother Gordon, had left her an annuity that yielded less than $100 a month. From time to time she accepted money from friends and relatives, and Mr. Fox recalls that she welcomed the old age pension of $40 a month when, on reaching the age of 70 in 1953, she became eligible to receive it. By October 1963, successive increases in the amount of that pension gave her an additional monthly income of $75.[2]

In her earlier years, the world of politics had not interested her to any degree. Her father, though he probably voted Conservative, was by no means partisan in politics, and at home she had never been exposed to lively political talk. True, while in New York, she had shared the excitement of the first days of the New Deal, but Canada was 'British soil' and different from 'the States'. Now at home again, however, the political ferment of the thirties was inescapable, and she found herself listening to "the prophetic voice" of J.S. Woodsworth. Shortly after her return to Toronto he had spoken to an audience of 10,000 in Massey Hall, and 'The Observer', describing the meeting on the editorial page of *The Toronto Daily Star*, wrote that the people of Canada at last were on the march. "A force of which Canadian politics for generations has known little is now at work. The invisible government of big interests is trembling on its throne".[3] Miss Dyke was intrigued by that idea, and she became an ardent supporter, if not a member of the Cooperative Commonwealth Federation (CCF), of which Mr. Woodsworth was the leader. Although the election of 1935 gave the party only seven seats in the House of Commons, it was a struggling minority that she could support, and in succeeding national elections she continued to vote CCF.

Toronto was the focus of her concern, however, and the 1934 report of the Lieutenant Governor's Commission on Housing Conditions was discouragingly reminiscent of Dr. Hastings' 1911 report on slum conditions in the city. Miss Dyke knew the organizations and agencies that had provided information for the Commission: the Local Council of Women, the Junior League, the Welfare Bureau, the Children's Aid Society, the Victorian Order of Nurses, the Visiting Homemakers' Association and the Social Service Department of the Toronto General Hospital. They had reported insanitation, inadequate water supply and lack of sanitary conveniences. The incidence of tuberculosis that she had seen diminishing was being reversed, and there was an increase in infant mortality. Juvenile delinquency and adult crime were on the rise, family life was disrupted and children neglected.[4] The vision of emerging social well-being she had shared with Dr. Hastings had been shattered. Poverty, the chief enemy in those days, still remained unvanquished, and its insidious tentacles had been multiplied by economic depression.[5]

Even the lower prices that enabled Miss Dyke to get along were suspect. Shortage of jobs was forcing workers to accept low wages that helped to keep prices down. That had been made clear in a report on labour conditions in Toronto industries that employed women needle workers.[6] It had been prepared by Winifred Hutchison who, at the request of the 1934 Price Spreads Enquiry, a parliamentary investigation of conditions in the retail trade, had been released from the staff of the National Council of the YWCA to undertake the task. She and her assistants had studied more than 50 firms most of which supplied large department stores. Interviewing employers, employees, trade union officials and officers of the Canadian Manufacturers' Association, they found that, in order to keep prices down, the stores were buying in large quantities in the cheapest market. This policy threatened Toronto manufacturers who were competing with similar industries in Quebec, where wages were even lower than in Toronto and manufactured goods cheaper. So it was that the workers, fearful of losing their jobs, were induced to accept pay so low that the researchers could not see how they were able to feed and clothe themselves. 'The Observer' of *The Toronto Daily Star* described the report as "a revelation of studied injustice, crafty meanness and callous inhumanity".[7] It was, in fact, all of that, a depressing account of women and girls working under intolerable pressure to fill rush orders, victims of devious evasions of minimun wage regulations and plagued with uncertainty about the amount of their earnings. Little wonder they suffered strain and fatigue! Moreover, although the environment in some of the factories was reasonably good if they were kept clean, there were others where overcrowding, poor ventilation, and inadequate lighting created additional health hazards.

Meanwhile in Toronto, radical political groups moving in to organize the unemployed created a rift in the CCF about which Miss Dyke may well have had ambivalent feelings. On May Day in 1936, this movement reached a peak when the CCF and the Communist Party jointly sponsored a parade through the city followed by a rally of 20,000 unemployed in the new Maple Leaf Gardens. Participants in the demonstration thought it an unqualified success, but the leaders of the CCF had recently adopted a policy of non-cooperation with the Communist Party, and to them it was an equally *unqualified* disaster.[8] Nevertheless, many of the rank and file of the CCF welcomed a 'united front'. Their enthusiasm had been aroused by accounts of burgeoning social and economic justice in the Soviet Union, ideas that captured Miss Dyke's enthusiasm. Mr. Woodsworth was her lodestar, however, and in the long run she remained loyal to CCF leadership. People who knew her even slightly in the late years of her life and who remember little else about her have not forgotten that "she was CCF". Yet she seemed to have retained a certain aura about the Soviet Union. A friend with whom she had occasional lively conversations recalls that she strongly disagreed with him when, shortly after the war, having just read Orwell's *Animal Farm*, he told her that he found it hilariously funny. "I loathe the book", she retorted and went on to say that the chief menaces to the world were the big impersonal international corporations. She told him, too, that someone in her personal past had shocked her by expressing the view that big American firms would take over Canada quite amicably. The friend's further comment is enlightening: "In spite of her personal experience of sin and sinners in the political world, she did not enjoy Orwell's take-off on Lenin, Stalin and Trotsky . . . perhaps she just thought I was too bourgeois and involved with a big impersonal corporation (a life insurance company)– i.e. you can't take our arguments too seriously".[9] Eunice had always liked to argue, and "a capitalist friend" with a sense of humour was an enticing adversary. Miss Dyke was nonetheless a genuine socialist. According to a niece, she even came to question whether she should have accepted a larger salary than her nurses in the Department of Public Health.

Through these trying years, her former nurse colleagues in the Department of Public Health, now in substantially smaller numbers, carried on as in the past. Wherever there was sickness, a public health nurse was there, but Miss Dyke, however much she may have wished it were possible, could no longer share in the development of the work in Toronto, a desire she expressed in writing to Dr. Hastings from Paris in May 1924. Nevertheless, she occasionally called on successive directors of the division of public health nursing, but, they, while respectful of her knowledge and foresight, were too busy for the prolonged conversations to which she was prone.

Changing Needs for Health Care

"I always admired how Miss Dyke left the past behind and began afresh," says Florence Emory. The new interest that increasingly absorbed her energies grew out of a conviction born of her experience in public health work that older people in the community had special needs that all too often were "swept under the rug". The impetus came from a group of elderly women living alone on city relief in "ill-furnished rooms with inadequate cooking, laundry and heating facilities". They had found refuge from cold and loneliness in the lounge of the YWCA in McGill Street. As their numbers grew, they took possession of the pleasant room, and young women, for whom, in fact, the YWCA existed, were being excluded. Finally, the YWCA Board had no choice but to ask the older women to leave. Alternative arrangements were made for them to meet at the House of Friendship (Carlton Street United Church), and members of the Business and Professional Women's Club agreed to take turns in meeting with them once a week. Miss Dyke first met this group on a Wednesday evening in 1935, when she was asked to substitute for a 'B and P' member who was unable to be present. The situation caught her interest, so she continued to join the group every week. Casual association was not enough for her, however. Gradually she succeeded in getting the addresses of those who attended the social times and had no difficulty in persuading members of the Business and Professional Women's Club to deliver a Christmas gift to each of them. Seemingly a 'lady bountiful' gesture, in Miss Dyke's thinking this was much more. She was convinced that loneliness was the greatest problem of the elderly and that ways must be found to encourage them to participate in meaningful activities.[10] Here was a group of women who in time might respond to such a challenge and, to test that possibility, she continued to work with them until they became the nucleus of the Second Mile Club, which she founded in 1937. It was the first organization of 'senior citizens' in Toronto, indeed in Canada !

Working with that small group of elderly women who had been evicted from the YWCA, Miss Dyke had caught a glimmer of a cause to be espoused. To alleviate the hardship of the unemployed or wipe out corrupt merchandising practices and unjust working conditions in industry would require political action that she could support but not initiate. She had, however, opted for a career with broader dimensions than at first she realized. Her immediate strategy was to interest organizations of influential women. Socialist though she was, she had no scruples about calling upon people, whether or not they shared her political convictions, to support the project that she envisaged. Thus, with the help of friends, she was able to persuade the Zonta Club, the Soroptimists and the Princess Elizabeth Chapter of the I.O.D.E. to share with the Business and Professional Women's Club responsibility for the social time, each for one Wednesday evening a month. When there were five Wednesdays, Miss Kathleen Cowan, a YWCA Board member who had continued to keep in touch with the group, entertained them in her home. As Miss Dyke organized this outreach, she kept in close touch with new developments. In the summer of 1936, she obtained a contribution from Joseph Atkinson, publisher of the *Toronto Daily Star* for street car and ferry tickets to take the women to the Island, and arranged picnics with them over there once a week. Tuesdays were picnic days, and on Thursdays the group met to sew at the office of the Neighbourhood Workers' Association in Wellesley Street.[11]

Notwithstanding their enjoyment of these activities, however, the group continued to resent having been evicted from the YWCA. Their hostility grew with the passing of time, until an imaginative librarian, Lillias Alexander, ('Dit' to her friends), who was in charge of the Downtown Branch of the Public Libraries, came up with the idea of taking them on a journey, "Round the World with Books". Many years later Miss Dyke recalled that the reading began with Nellie McClung in the Canadian west and went on with the adventures of Anne Morrow Lindberg over the Arctic. It then proceeded by stages she had forgotten to the beauty of a small island off the coast of Ireland in Maurice O'Sullivan's story, *Twenty Years A-Growing*. Miss Dyke shared the enchantment of this glimpse of the world of books and, with a tinge of hyperbole, she described in retrospect the effect on the women: "The esprit de corps of this group was based on . . . hatred and malice. Under Miss Alexander's magic touch, they became participating citizens with dreams and a sense of adventure".[12]

The experience confirmed her conviction that broadened horizons help to dispel loneliness and give life fresh meaning. Shortly arrangements were made for the group to have the use of rooms on the second floor of the Occupational Therapy workshop in Bloor Street West every afternoon. At that location, on 17 March 1937, (Kathleen Cowan's birthday), the Second Mile Club was organized with Lady Falconer as President. A board of directors was named, a statement of membership policy adopted, and an auditor appointed. They chose the name, Second Mile Club, not in the scriptural sense of the reference in St. Matthew 5:41 but, as Miss Dyke explained, because members of the Club were 60 years of age or more and, now released from earlier responsibilities, were ready to move into a new phase of living. The program of the group had already taken shape, and Miss Dyke had been sending weekly reports of activities and developments to a committee comprised of Kathleen Cowan and three interested social workers. Now she continued in the leadership role working with the new board of directors and was paid 'a salary' of five dollars a month. More adequate accommodation was acquired in Scadding House, Trinity Square, and the Club was open to members all day every day but Sunday.

The Second Mile Club had always had only women members, but, when it was learned that Scadding House would be needed for other purposes, and new quarters must be found, consideration was given to a merger with the all male Good Neighbours Club which had also had accommodation in Scadding House. The latter had been organized for unemployed men during the depression and, although, with the outbreak of war, many of the men had enlisted, there were still some who wished to continue their association. In the end, it was decided that the two clubs would not unite but that, if any of the men were interested in joining the Second Mile Club, they should feel free to do so, and from then on men were welcomed as members. Meanwhile, alternative accommodation must be found. The members, resentful of the Club having to be moved so often, were eager to have a centre where they could go whenever they wanted to. What rejoicing then, when in 1940, a four-roomed apartment in St.

Nicholas Street was acquired for their use! Now, with kitchen facilities, it was possible to cook a simple meal, and for the first time Miss Dyke had an office. Previously, although she often spent full days at the Club, she had done the executive work from her home. In the new centre there was also a hostess, a versatile lady who always wore a hat. Each morning, Miss Dyke and she reviewed the plans for the day which the hostess recorded briefly, adding also her own activities of the day before. They were manifold. She not only received visitors but found time to talk with members; she presided over tea parties and occasional luncheons, did the Club shopping, helped with handicrafts and sometimes attended meetings to represent the Club.

The centre was pleasantly informal. Several times a week, three or four members would join in preparing their supper, each contributing either an item of food or a share of the cost. This spirit of comradeship reached out to new-comers, who came in growing numbers. Typical of the many who turned up was a shy little woman who timidly set foot over the doorstep and sidled into a chair. Day after day she did this until she was sure enough of herself and others to join two or three members who sat chatting at a nearby table. They welcomed her, and from then on she belonged. Gradually too, the self-absorption of individuals gave way to feeling for others' misfortunes. There was a Scotsman who, though counting on his wife's eventual release from a mental hospital, was obliged to give up their home. When other members learned of his dilemma, the Club arranged to store his furniture instead of him having to sell it. Further evidence of growing confidence occurred when the Princess Elizabeth Chapter of the I.O.D.E., which had shared in early efforts to carry on monthly programs, wanted to give a party for the Club. Miss Dyke, who was opposed to having things done for the elderly, consulted the members. They decided to reverse the role, and the result was a delightful party for the I.O.D.E., hosted by the Second Mile Club.[13]

The proportion of older men and women in Toronto's population was growing rapidly, and more and more of them, having heard of the Second Mile Club, sought it out as a place where they would find others of similar age and interests. This influx was encouraged by organizations and individuals who were convinced that the Club had become an

212

essential service to the elderly, and it was not long until the membership had outgrown the apartment in St. Nicholas Street. Plainly, if the Club were to continue, a search for more adequate premises must be undertaken. Several places were considered before Janet Nielson, Miss Dyke's former colleague in the Department of Public Health, discovered a fine old house at 192 Carlton Street that was for sale. Surely here was an ideal home for the Club. Its fourteen rooms would provide for larger numbers immediately and also accommodate future growth. It was in the midst of a rooming-house district that housed the largest proportion of Toronto's old people who lived alone, and it was on a streetcar line that would bring people in from all parts of the city until neighbourhood centres could be developed. The sale price was $22,000.00, reasonable enough for such a house set in a spacious lot: 30 metres frontage by 68 metres deep. But the Second Mile Club had no money. Moreover, the house would need structural changes that would add considerably to the cost.

Miss Dyke concluded, and the Board of Directors agreed with her, that the only recourse was to ask the City to purchase the property and let it to the Club at a nominal annual rental. This would require an application to the Board of Control, but how was it to be done? Shades of past humiliation lingered in Miss Dyke's mind. Nevertheless, she set about planning a strategy. The Club had many friends: voluntary organizations that had supported it from the early days, visiting nurses, church and social workers in the downtown area, and the Visiting Homemakers' Association, of which she was still a committee member. She was also certain of the backing of the Toronto Welfare Council which was organizing a Division of Old Age, the name of which she had suggested. Further, the United Welfare Chest, although it had no funds for capital expenditures such as the purchase of property, would guarantee a yearly operating budget. The Chest was an outgrowth of the United Welfare Fund which, since 1940, had combined the fund-raising efforts of 18 established organizations. Additional agencies were admitted to membership in the Chest to make possible cooperative fund-raising and coordinated planning. In 1947, the name was changed to Community Chest and is now the United Appeal. The Second Mile Club was accepted as a member of the Chest in 1947. A canvas of the churches in the area: St. Peter's Anglican and the two United Churches, Sherbourne Street and St. Andrew's, brought favourable response, and also promising was the prospect that the Second Mile Club might have "a friend at court". Mrs. Mary Ann Somerville, one of the Directors, who was a friend of Controller H.E. McCallum, undertook to acquaint him with the purpose of the Club, its history and current program and the need for more adequate premises.

A careful brief was prepared, explaining all the circumstances, including the fact that for ten years the Second Mile Club had conducted the only recreational centre for the increasing population of older people in Toronto. Then on 11 September 1946, Miss Mabel Stoakley, President of the Club's Board of Directors, with the support of a large deputation from various welfare and social organizations, presented the brief to the Board of Control. Miss Bessie Touzel, Executive Secretary of the United Welfare Chest, assured the Board of the Chest's guarantee of an operating budget and urged favourable consideration of the application. Controller McCallum, whom Mrs. Somerville had convinced of the importance of the Club, had already discussed the matter with the City's Director of Recreation, and on his motion it was referred to the appropriate officials in order to obtain an estimate of the probable cost and to look into the City's legal position in the matter. As a result of these enquiries, on 16 October, the Board of Control recommended to the City Council that the property be purchased by the City, and made suitable for the purposes of the Second Mile Club at an estimated cost of $36,500, and leased to the Club at a rental of $1.00 a year. However, the transaction was subject to the approval of the Ontario Department of Municipal Affairs and the City Solicitor was instructed to apply for authority to proceed.[14] To meet the legal requirements, the Club was obliged to draw up a formal constitution as a basis for incorporation. Finally, on 2 June 1947, Letters Patent were issued to confirm an Ontario Government Charter for the Second Mile Club as "a corporation without share capital".[15] During the summer renovations were carried out and preparations made for the move which climaxed in a large opening reception in September.

Meanwhile, Miss Dyke had made known that she planned to resign in the near future, but she was appointed "acting executive director" as from 1 July 1947. Additional staff included Susie Dickinson, her secretary, and Frances Hogg, the lady with the hat, as member hostess.[16] The new centre was open all day every day, and, with the help of devoted volunteers, the program was carried on much as in the past except that now there was adequate space for meetings as well as crafts and games. There was also a kitchen that made possible more extensive hospitality. There has never been any doubt of the wisdom of the action taken to bring about the move to 192 Carlton Street, where the Second Mile Club still operates a centre, now one of five in Metropolitan Toronto, (Carlton, East Toronto, High Park, North Toronto and Rotary-Laughlen), as well as a visiting service for members who are confined to their homes. Again, Miss Dyke, having recognized an emerging need in a changing society, had made a unique contribution to Canadian life.

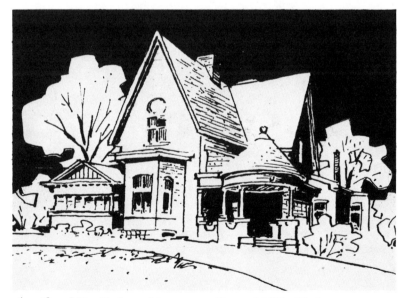

Another Miss Dyke achievement: Second Mile Club

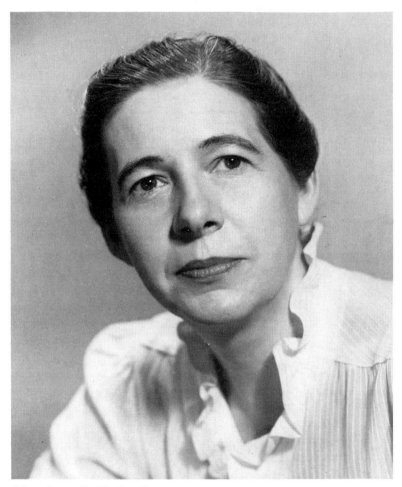

Mrs. Jean Good, October 1946

Chapter Thirteen

A New Way of Life

In the City and in the Country

Miss Dyke, now past 60, had been thinking for some-time about retirement and whether she was ready for "a new phase of living". First, however, she would have liked to have found someone she could trust to succeed her in the Second Mile Club and to carry on her concerns for the ageing. Then one Sunday in April 1946, sitting in church and only half listening to the sermon, she took special note of a young woman who always sat with her two children in the next pew but whom she knew only slightly. Jean Good, the woman in question, was the widow of a Baptist minister who had died only seven years after their marriage. Miss Dyke had recognized strength of purpose in the woman's movements and had heard the lilt in her voice when she spoke to her children or to friends who greeted her. She had kind eyes that shone with merriment, and the lines around her mouth were marks of the courage that overcomes unspoken grief. Miss Dyke could hardly wait until the service ended to tell the young woman what she had in mind, and with only a discreet pause after the benediction, invited her to go home with her for lunch.

Mrs. Good hesitated. At work all week, she looked forward to Sunday as a day with her children, but Miss Dyke's insistence was irresistible. She accepted the invitation, and over a simple meal in the apartment in Hazelton Avenue, she listened to Miss Dyke's description of the Second Mile Club and her ideas about what must be done to give dignity and meaning to life in the later years. She believed that modern living was robbing the elderly of self-esteem.

They were lonely, often estranged from their families, their needs ignored by the helping professions. Doctors would say to a patient, "What can you expect at your age?" Social workers were too often victims of an ultra-professionalism that created stereotypes of the elderly and how they should be treated. Her concern was not for the poor only. There were many men and women of ample means whose lives were equally impaired.

Then Miss Dyke turned to the future. The proportion of elderly in the population was increasing rapidly, and without further delay, steps must be taken to ensure for them the sense of well-being so essential to a meaningful role in society. It was not a matter of doing things *for* them but of enabling them to do things for themselves and others. They should have suitable housing in a community where they belonged. Services such as visiting homemakers (meals on wheels had not yet been heard of) should be available so they could live in their own homes as long as possible. When they could no longer manage alone, there should be well-run group homes for them, with nursing care if needed. "A neglected segment of society," she said, "affects the whole." There should be opportunities for further education, formal as well as informal, to widen their horizons. If they needed or wanted to work for pay, they should not be excluded from the labour market. Surely there were jobs they could do better than young people, not in spite of their age but as a result of age and experience. The same applied to voluntary work in the community, and suitable possibilities for such service should be opened up for them. She believed in the advantages of being older, and she thought that what senior citizens could do for the community should have as much attention as what the community could do for them.

Jean Good listened with rapt attention, saying little as the hours flitted by and, as she looks back on that experience now, she speaks with conviction when she says, "Miss Dyke was far ahead of her time".

Miss Dyke had thought of Mrs. Good as a candidate for leadership of the Second Mile Club, but that kind of work did not appeal to her. She was more interested in the broad dimensions of the needs of the elderly. She had spent the war years on the staff of the War-time Prices and Trade Board, working from the Toronto office on the enforcement of rental

218

regulations and was well acquainted with housing in the city and the conditions in which many elderly people lived. That activity was now winding down, and she had decided to resign. But before looking for a new job, she planned to go to California for a niece's wedding. Miss Dyke intimated that the Toronto Welfare Council was looking for a full-time secretary for the new Division on Old Age. That sounded interesting to Mrs. Good, and Miss Dyke lost no time. The next day, though unaware that Jean Good had a background in social work, she called on Miss Touzel, Executive Secretary of the Council, to recommend her as a promising candidate for the new job. The appointment was made, and Mrs. Good began work as Secretary of the Division on Old Age of the Toronto Welfare Council of the Community Chest of Greater Toronto. Designation of the post in the Minutes of a meeting of the Directors of the Second Mile Club that Mrs. Good attended on 16 June 1946, was so enticing that she did not go to California. She kept in close touch with Miss Dyke during the remaining years of the latter's life, and found her a stimulating mentor whom she could depend upon. Miss Dyke returned that trust, and they became firm friends. "We were working in the field of geriatrics," says Mrs. Good, "before we knew the meaning of the word." [1]

The autumn days of 1947 were prosperous for the Club. The atmosphere was informal. New members came, and Miss Dyke as leader and Director was at her best, but she had not wavered from her decision to retire. In January, at the request of the Board of Directors, she agreed to remain until a new executive director had been selected, and finally on 5 March, John A. Falconbridge, B.A., B.S.W., was appointed at an annual salary of $3,000, his duties to begin 1 April 1948.[2] The choice disappointed Miss Dyke. Her candidate was Paul Joliffe, another recent social work graduate, who she thought was more in tune with the spirit and purpose of the Club. A majority of the Board voted against him, however, supporting one of the Directors who opposed the appointment because Mr. Joliffe's brother was a CCF member of the Ontario Legislature, a fact that in Miss Dyke's eyes, might well have been in his favour.

The Board granted her two months' leave of absence with pay from 1 April until 31 May, a courtesy for which she thanked the Board of Directors in a letter read when they met on 12 May 1948. That was her last personal involvement with the Second Mile Club, but her concern for the well-being of the elderly had by no means ended. She was in constant touch with Jean Good, "always brimming with ideas," says Jean, who also speaks of having frequently turned to her for advice when faced with perplexing situations. Both women were members of the Visiting Home-makers' Committee, and both urged the extension of service to older people to enable them to remain in their own homes. Miss Dyke's persistence in the matter was irritating to Elizabeth Dewitt, Executive Secretary of the Association, who still remembers with regret altercations that occurred. She herself was equally convinced of the needs of the elderly but was hampered by a budget already overtaxed with calls to help families with young children, who were coping with emergencies. Miss Dyke, in her enthusiasm, would brook no obstacles, however, and her tenacity became irksome to those who did not share her vision. Jean Good, on the other hand, who did share her vision, had such confidence in her integrity and creative energy that she never wavered in her appreciation of the older woman. To Miss Dyke, who had felt betrayed in other professional relationships, Mrs. Good was heir to her concern. Their mutual understanding was unassailable.

During these later years, Miss Dyke found other friends who, like Jean Good, gave her a new lease on life. While the Second Mile Club was still in St. Nicholas Street, she had come into touch with an English couple, Doreen and Cecil Corps,[3] who lived in Brown Hill, a village in a swampy unproductive area near Lake Simcoe, halfway between Sutton and Mount Albert. Mrs. Corps, as 'Mary Star', editor of an advice column in the *Toronto Daily Star* dealt with floods of letters, many of them from older people who wrote of loss of friends of their own age. They were lonely, and she, having heard of the Second Mile Club, often suggested it as a place of congenial companionship. Then one day Miss Dyke telephoned her to ask her please not to send any more people. She explained that the apartment in St. Nicholas Street was already "bursting at the seams", and, to their great regret, they could not accept any more members or even visitors. "But," she added, "would you care to come in one day and see the people and place for yourself?" Mrs. Corps accepted the invitation, and that first meeting of the two women was the beginning of a mutually enriching friendship that never wavered through Miss Dyke's remaining years.

Miss Dyke believed that life for the elderly need not be solemn and dull any more than for the young, and both Doreen Corps and her husband, Cec, agreed with her ideas. They became interested in the Second Mile Club, and Cec was soon one of the most active volunteers. "He and a Mrs. Handly from Kleinburg worked together, Miss Dyke holding the reins," recalls Doreen. With Mrs. Handly playing the piano and Cec. his violin, the members had many a good sing-song, and "God bless this house" became the 'home song' of the Club. While Miss Dyke was incontestably in charge, she was never aloof from the members. There was a party shortly after the move to Carlton Street when she persuaded them all to put on old fashioned nightcaps that had come down to her from her family. Everybody looked so absurd that selfconsciousness melted in mirth, and everybody had a good time.

Jean Good remembers that there were both social workers and nurses who were *not amused* by such antics, but the Corps, themselves blest with a sense of humour, shared Miss Dyke's sense of the absurd. Her delight in a humorous situation is one of Doreen's most vivid recollections of the woman. Of all Doreen's stories, however, none rivals one that Janet Holmes tells. Although Miss Dyke was a frequent guest in the Holmes' home, Janet had never seen her apartment and was delighted to be invited to tea with one of her best friends as a companion. Not a detail of the living-room escaped the notice of the two teen-agers, and they were taken aback to find several books by Ethel M. Dell on one of the tables. "They were novels," chuckles Janet, "like the Harlequin ones of today." Her friend and she had read them, but that they might interest Miss Dyke boggled the imagination. Sensing their dismay, she quipped, "That's how I get my romance".

The fact that Eunice Dyke had never married occasioned frequent comment. Some people thought it was because she resented men in general, plainly a specious explanation for she enjoyed the friendship of numbers of men. More probably, however, like many other professional women of her time, she was so absorbed in her work that marriage, with the care of a family, seemed irrelevant. Moreover in these years, she found a family home with the Corps whom she often visited in Brown Hill, and they, in turn, discovered a different person under the martinet exterior that other people talked about.

The Corps had moved to Brown Hill during the Depression. Married in 1929, they had furnished a new home in Toronto and settled in happily. Then Cec lost his job. Without too much difficulty he found another but shortly lost it too, and they decided "to hole in" and spend the rest of the Depression in the country. Much searching led them to the house in Brown Hill which they rented for four dollars a month. It was primitive living, without either electricity or indoor plumbing, but they had a garden and kept chickens. Brown Hill was a totally new experience for them. Their neighbours reminded them of Kentucky Hill people they had read about. Feckless and roughly spoken, they were despised by the respectable citizens of Sutton and Mount Albert. Nevertheless, the three villages did have one thing in common. They were all "crazy about baseball", and Brown Hill had a consuming ambition to have a team that would qualify for the Sutton-Mount Albert league. At first the Corps seemed suspiciously respectable, but initial hostility gradually wore off, and they were accepted, one might even say, invaded. There were two doors in their kitchen, one opening to the east and one to the west, and as time went on, one group would be leaving by the west door as a new crowd came in through the one to the east. One day a deputation came more formally to ask Cec to coach their baseball team. Taken aback, he explained that he didn't know a thing about baseball. Nobody played the game in England where he had grown up. "You can read, can't you!" they retorted. "Here's a book that will tell you everything you need to know about it." Cec relented, studied the book and together they built up a team that was admitted to the league, but they never did win a game.

Living among the Brown Hill people, the Corps became aware that, in face of privation, many of them, especially some of the women, were resourceful and courageous, and Doreen thought that people in Toronto should know about Brown Hill. She began to write occasional letters to the *Toronto Daily Star*, describing daily life and incidents that aroused her admiration. One episode that she recalls was the premature birth of an infant when the local midwife who delivered the child used the oven as an incubator. Without either a doctor or a hospital in the vicinity, which they could not have afforded in any case, the people were 'making do'. At the time, the newspaper was looking for someone to edit a new advice column, and, recognizing the facile pen of a compassionate woman, asked Doreen to take on the job. She refused until one day when Cec was away and she had put on an old pair of his overalls to go out to feed the chickens, a shiny black Buick drove up. A well dressed man with a large package under his arm came into the yard, and asked, "Are you by any chance, Mrs. Corps?" Assured of her identity, he explained that the *Toronto Daily Star* would like very much to have her edit the column. She could begin at once using the pen-name, 'Mary Star'. He had even brought a package of paper. Half reluctantly she agreed, and she and her husband rented a room in Gould Street in Toronto that gave them a *pied à terre* in the city. Thus opened up the series of events that led to Mrs. Doreen Corps' meeting with Eunice Dyke, who later became so much a part of their life.

Life in the Corps household in Brown Hill was never either solemn or dull. For Miss Dyke it was a second home. She was fond of Cec. Says Doreen, "He called her gal and managed her, and she liked it". A third member of the household was Norman Green, an actor and producer at Hart House Theatre, who often had no money and had come to live with the Corps. Miss Dyke enjoyed knowing him, too, and she tried not to miss any plays he was involved in. In Doreen who, like Jean Good, understood her and trusted her implicitly, she found a dearly loved friend. She was the only person Doreen ever allowed to read the letters to 'Mary Star'. "Miss Dyke often helped me answer them. She seemed to understand what the people wanted," Doreen recalled. She also helped with the housework, her favourite chore cleaning the coal-oil lamps. Once she took as her project the clearing up and cleaning of the cellar, a task Doreen dreaded and had tended to put off. The only trouble was that Doreen was a hoarder, and Miss Dyke wanted to throw out things she was sure the Corps would never use. Helping with the cooking was another of Miss Dyke's pastimes. Since she had had her own apartment, she had taken up cooking in earnest for the first time in her life, and she enjoyed it. She collected recipes of all sorts and liked to try them out on the Corps. Doreen remembers Cec's story of an acrimonious discussion of what he liked to eat. At the time he was teaching in the 'school train' that went to places in Northern Ontario where there were no schools, and Doreen had gone to England to visit relatives and friends. Knowing that he would be going home for a few days, Doreen suggested that he invite Miss Dyke and two women whom they knew who lived in Mount Albert to come for a visit. Both Miss Dyke and one of the Mount Albert ladies were sure they knew Cec's tastes, but Miss Dyke usually came out on top in their arguments. "The stuff that Miss Dyke gave Cec to eat! It was awful", the Mount Albert friends later told Doreen. However, Cec was prepared for anything; Miss Dyke had once made him a cup of hot chocolate with buttermilk.

Up in Brown Hill, Miss Dyke by no means limited herself to the Corps household. Life in the village fascinated her. Most of all she enjoyed the baseball games. For hours on end she would watch the play, cheering for the winning side and urging on the losers. She found time to visit the women and knew the homes where there were new babies. She loved the children and knew them all by name. Like Doreen, she admired the skill and resourcefulness of the local midwife who lived a busy life in her own household in addition to the nursing duties that fell to her lot. Talking with her, Miss Dyke recognized the importance of midwifery in the village. Here was fresh light on a subject that had not come to her attention for many years. Back in 1916 midwifery had been an issue before the Canadian National Association of Trained Nurses, and although there is no record of her opinion in the matter, it is unlikely that she would have rejected the consensus of the Association. Following the lead of the medical profession, the nurses believed that midwives, lacking the skills and knowledge of the trained nurse, could be the cause of many deaths in childbirth. In Brown Hill that idea lost validity. Nurses had been concerned to establish their own profession but had they at the same time ignored the needs of countless people who could not afford professional services or were too remote to have access to them?[4] It was a nagging question. Doreen remembers her often saying, "Life up here is an epic". It was an epic with many themes.

Most of her friends and relatives in the city would not have recognized the Eunice Dyke of Brown Hill. She surprised even the Corps. Yet she was still 'the head nurse'. She rearranged the pots and pans in Doreen's kitchen until Doreen called a halt because she could never find the one she wanted, but Miss Dyke still insisted that her arrangement was better balanced. Then there was her passion for getting rid of things not in use. Once Doreen asked her to bring a dress from the room in Gould Street up to Brown Hill, but, instead of picking up the one she had come for, she went through the wardrobe and took out several dresses to be discarded. "Mrs. Corps never wears these," she told the landlady. When she had gone, the landlady put them back where they belonged, fortunately, for one of them was Doreen's favourite summer dress.

Doreen took no umbrage at these eccentricities. To her they were minor matters that they could laugh about together. Nevertheless, from time to time she was taken aback at things Miss Dyke would say or do. She insisted, for instance, that Doreen was trying to domesticate Cec because she expected him to help with household chores. One day she chided Doreen for arranging the appointment for a painful dental operation at a time when she knew Cec would not be free to go with her. "I thought I was protecting him from unnecessary misery", Doreen recalled, but Miss Dyke had told her that she had robbed him of an experience he should have had a chance to go through with his wife. Nor could Doreen get used to Miss Dyke's habit of going through the desk of her secretary (when she had one) to check whether the young woman had completed her work. Doreen thought this an invasion of privacy, but Miss Dyke justified it as a way of measuring competence: perhaps a hangover from the strict discipline of her training as a nurse, Doreen thought. Miss Dyke sometimes mentioned that strait-jacket and its effect on her, but she also talked to Doreen and to Jean Good about the unforgettable days she had spent in the Johns Hopkins Training School and the wisdom and foresight of her instructors. She felt that the experience she had had there and what she had learned about nursing should be recorded for posterity, but later, when friends went to see her, equipped with a tape recorder, she was unable to go through

225

with it. Although they remember the incident, they have never understood her hesitation unless, much older by then, she may have been intimidated by the mechanical recorder and missed the personal response of conversation.

While Miss Dyke went so often to Brown Hill and sometimes stayed as long as a week with the Corps, she also lived a full life in Toronto, and the Corps became a part of that too. They visited her often at her Hazelton Avenue apartment and also later at the Julia Greenshields Home on University Avenue where she lived from 1957 to 1964. Eunice Dyke's roots in Toronto were deep. She had many friends in the city as well as a considerable number of relatives, and she liked to keep in touch with them. Jean Good was one of those closest to her in these years, and she and Doreen (who after Cecil's death, married Carl Nolan and is now living in Tucson, Arizona), still enjoy reminiscing about 'Miss Dyke'. "She begged us to call her Eunice, but Cec and I could never bring ourselves to use her first name," explained Doreen, and Jean Good felt the same way about that degree of intimacy.

Past friends of Miss Dyke whom neither of the younger women ever knew often came into her conversation with them. One who stands out vividly in Doreen's mind was Elizabeth Nainby, an Englishwoman who had joined the staff of Havergal College in 1899 as a teacher of English and Mistress of the Boarding School. She retired in 1937, and that year's edition of *Laudamus*, the school magazine, told of her departure: "Miss Nainby, beloved by all the girls, past and present, left us this October for England after nearly forty years' work for the school she loved". One of Miss Dyke's most cherished possessions was a lovely brass kettle that Miss Nainby gave her as a memento of their friendship. Miss Dyke had always admired the sheen of its polish and the artistry of its design, and it brought back pleasant memories of having tea with Miss Nainby in her rooms at the College. Eventually she gave the kettle to Doreen who still treasures it in her home in Tucson, one of the few things she took with her when she left Canada.

Miss Dyke introduced the Corps to numbers of her friends and relatives, many of whom they would probably not otherwise have known. Doreen remembers, for instance, two contemporaries of Miss Dyke, Barbara Robertson, a New

Zealander, and Kate Miles, who had been 'Bride Brodie' of a column in *The Mail and Empire*,[5] chiefly because of frequent altercations between Mrs. Robertson and Miss Dyke. Mrs. Robertson was married to Irving Robertson, a son of John Ross Robertson, who was the founder of Toronto's Hospital for Sick Children. Mrs. Robertson, then Barbara Mackenzie, who had come to Canada in 1931, was an advocate of natural child birth, midwifery and well-baby nursing; she had founded The Canadian Mothercraft Society. Despite common interests, however, the two strong-minded women argued incessantly. Eunice Dyke had always thrived on argument, and there were differences in approach to the well-being of mothers and their babies that may have sparked dispute and led on to wrangling over personal matters. Perhaps, also, Miss Dyke's 'new light' on midwifery may have needed the fuel of controversy. In any case, Doreen recalls that when a dispute became overheated, Kate Miles would move in to restore 'the peace'.

Among the relatives, Doreen remembers most clearly Miss Dyke's beloved Aunt Tina – Christine Ryrie – wife of her mother's brother Harry. Other favourites were the Chisholms. James Ryrie's daughter Grace had married Brock Chisholm, and talk with them was unfailingly stimulating. Miss Dyke took pride in the family relationship with the Chisholms, and Brock's thinking left its mark on her. He was a physician and a psychiatrist who, after a few years in private practice, had a distinguished career in the Canadian Army and then as a civil servant in the field of health, both national and international. He was largely responsible for the Constitution of the World Health Organization of which he was the first Director General, and his dedication to preventive medicine and public health gave Miss Dyke international perspective on concerns that dominated her life. Dr. Chisholm was also identified with the cause of world peace. Service as a young man in the 1914-18 war and his later professional experience during and after the conflict of 1939 to 1945 had left him without illusions about war – what it had done and what it had not done– and he turned to a serious search for peace. This too was a matter that Miss Dyke had thought about a great deal. The key to Dr. Chisholm's influence on her and many others was, however, the kind of person he was – in the words of Anne

Winslow of the Carnegie Endowment for International Peace "a totally impartial human being... of no arrogance only a tremendous puritan conscience". Miss Dyke would have endorsed Miss Winslow's further comment that he seemed to function as a touchstone and bring out the best in people who were 'quite good' and sometimes to cause those not so good to show their worst. Besides, as John Grierson, founder of the National Film Board of Canada, observed, he had a native talent for teaching, "He went to the heart of a matter, saw it simply and said it well".[6]

Doreen also remembers Miss Dyke's sister, Mrs. Fox, as a "lovely looking woman and an attractive personality". She, of course, never knew the older sister, Mrs. West, who had died in 1930, but she does recall the hospitality of the West's home on the Scarborough Bluffs. There she met Ethel's daughter, Jean, who, after her mother's death, was her father's hostess and support. It was there, too, that the Corps became acquainted with R. Watson McLaine, a legendary figure who died in 1961 at the age of 94. His summer place was next to the West property, and his wife, who died well before him, was a sister of Joseph West. Through this connection, Miss Dyke had known him as 'Uncle Wat', the name later adopted for him by his Rotary friends and everybody else who knew him. Having looked after his mother and other elderly relatives for a large part of his life, Uncle Wat was concerned about the needs of older people. Miss Dyke found in him a kindred spirit who was hospitable to her ideas, and she interested him in the Second Mile Club, of which he became a lifelong supporter. Having no heir (first his wife had died and then his only son had died of leukemia at 55), as a memorial to his wife, he left property to the City of Toronto for a park that senior citizens might enjoy. On land that he owned, there is now the Rosetta McLaine Home for Senior Citizens as well as the park, Rosetta Gardens. Furthermore, the $300,000 residue of his estate, which he willed to the Rotary Club, helped to build Rotary Laughlen Centre, a home for Senior citizens in downtown Toronto, where the headquarters of the Second Mile Club is now housed.[7]

Miss Dyke's liveliness of mind was undiminished in these years of association with the Corps. Wherever she was, she read the newspaper daily and kept up-to-date on public affairs. Few things gave her more pleasure than political discussion, and says Doreen, "She always had an opinion". Her interest in the CCF had never flagged, and she especially admired Andrew Brewin. From 1943, when he first ran as a CCF candidate for the House of Commons until he was elected as member for Greenwood, Toronto, in 1962, she supported him in every way she could. Nor did she forget him then; his career in Parliament was one of her abiding interests.

Participation in organizations that interested her was another of her preoccupations. Still enthusiastic about Visiting Homemaker Service, she nevertheless, gave priority to the Division on Old Age of the Toronto Welfare Council. Although she never held office in the Committee of the Division, she was a staunch and loyal member and more often than not, led in the shaping of policy. She also belonged to the Canadian Association of Social Workers, which did not yet restrict membership to professional social workers, and meetings of the Toronto branch gave her a forum to air her conviction about cooperation among the helping professions, especially social work and public health nursing. With equal vigour, she criticized social workers' treatment of the elderly. Oblivious of the passing of time, she would talk on and on about these and other subjects that she thought needed attention. Many members came to look upon her as a doddering old woman who talked too much. Yet those who remember her acknowledge that her ideas were sound, and that they would have done well to listen and act on them. In fact, a few individuals began shortly to speak out on the question of cooperation. In February 1968, Margaret Reynolds, supervisor of Hospital Health Service in the Nursing Division of the Department of Public Health, and Kathleen Gow, who had directed medical social service in the Hospital for Sick Children, co-authored an article "Public Health Nurse and Social Worker– Partners or Adversaries?" that was published in the February issue of *Canadian Journal of Public Health*.

Not all of her habitual associations continued to hold Miss Dyke's interest however. In the middle fifties she severed her lifelong connection with the Baptist denomination. She had become disenchanted with Park Road Baptist Church of which she had been a member since its inception.

As an off-shoot of the Jarvis Street Church that had replaced Bond Street Baptist Church to which her Ryrie grandparents had belonged, it had deep roots for her. The Jarvis Street Church, after the appointment of the Rev. T.T. Shields as its pastor in 1910, had become a centre of theological controversy. A fiery fundamentalist, Shields attacked the alleged modernism of McMaster University, where Baptist ministers were educated, and precipitated a long period of strife within the Baptist Denomination in Canada. He would brook no opposition, and, in 1922, members who could neither accept his theology nor endure his personality were evicted. Some of them joined the Walmer Road Baptist Church, and a larger number, of whom Miss Dyke was one, formed the Central Baptist Church holding services for the time being in Castle Memorial Hall of McMaster University.[8] In 1927, they moved into a newly built church in Park Road and changed the name of the congregation. A quarter of a century later, when the congregation was well established, Miss Dyke became aware of a group she thought were trying to get control of the congregation by favouring more affluent members and ignoring people of lesser means. According to Ben Holmes, there were probably several episodes that she might have objected to, but this one was the 'last straw'. She renounced her membership and began to attend the weekly meetings of the Society of Friends. Quaker opposition to war and dedication to peace attracted her; she found the new association congenial, and 17 April 1955, she joined the Society of Friends in Toronto. She frequently spoke in 'meeting' expressing ideas that Friends who remember her describe as having invariably given them food for thought.

Eunice Dyke had friends in the Quaker community whom she had known for many years, among them Violet Carroll, the public health nurse who had travelled across Canada by C.P.R. with returned soldiers who were recuperating from influenza after the first world war. Violet and two sisters, born 'Quakers', lived in the family home in the east end of Toronto, and during Miss Dyke's remaining active years, she was a frequent guest in the Carroll household. On Sundays she would go home from 'meeting' with the sisters and after lunch, resting on a sofa in the sun porch, she would talk with Violet about the early days in the Nursing Division. These conversations cemented their friendship. Miss Carroll had supported her in the controversy over Miss Bullick's dismissal, but the intervening years had not blotted out her questioning of some aspects of Miss Dyke's conduct in the affair. She especially resented the calling of a meeting of the nurses at Nora Moore's home which she felt had embarrassed Miss Moore who had already been appointed to succeed Miss Dyke. More significant, in Miss Carroll's recollection, however, was Miss Dyke's ability as an administrator and a teacher from whom she had learned what it meant to be a public health nurse and who had inspired her to try to be one of the best,[9] which, in the opinion of her colleagues, she became.

Eunice had a third bout with cancer in 1958 and spent several weeks in hospital, returning afterward to the Julia Greenshields Home, where she was living in 1960, when the Canadian Public Health Association, at its Jubilee Meeting in Halifax, awarded to her 'in absentia' an Honorary Life Membership for devoted service to public health. The citation, published in the July issue of the *Canadian Journal of Public Health*, singled out two achievements: "the development of generalized public health nursing service, introduced through the foresight and energy of Miss Dyke and Dr. C.J.O.C. Hastings", *and* the establishing of close liaison between public health and associated community welfare and social services. Still another celebration of her accomplishments occurred on her 80th birthday, 26 February 1963, when a reception arranged in her honour through the Second Mile Club, brought together men and women who had encouraged and supported her work in establishing the Club as a viable service. Facing the trials of old age, she enjoyed these honours that bespoke the achievements of a lifetime.[10]

Chapter Fourteen

Her Last Days

As years passed by, old age undermined her stamina. Dread of the return of cancer haunted her. In 1966 she spent a period in hospital for a series of tests but there was no evidence of another flare-up of the disease. Nevertheless, she had failed not only physically but also mentally, and her tendency to take charge was undiminished, so she had become a problem for the management of the Julia Greenshields Home. To avoid further clashes, the Director told her relatives that, on her release from hospital, it would not be possible to have Miss Dyke return. The Home had no infirmary, and they were preparing to move to a new building on St. Clair Avenue West, where there would be no provision for the nursing care that she would soon need. At the time, there were few nursing homes for the elderly in Toronto and to find a suitable one proved difficult. Ironically, she who had so clearly discerned the future need of such institutions, was now a victim of lack of foresight on the part of the community. Finally, her niece, Jean West, and nephew, John Fox, discovered 'Twin Elms' on Keele Street, near Steeles Avenue, a remote location in the 1960's and a very long way from Miss Dyke's accustomed neighbourhood. Nothing more promising being available, she was moved there in the spring.

Friends who went to see her at 'Twin Elms' were grieved by evidences of her failing mental powers. Because most of the other patients were senile, some of her friends thought that in a more stimulating atmosphere, she would not have deteriorated so rapidly. Whether or not they were right is a moot question. The decline of mental faculties is a perplexing phenomenon. She no longer lived in the future but seemed not to be unhappy in the present. She spoke of her fellow patients as 'my people', and until she was bedridden, went each morning after breakfast to the office of the Director to tell him what should be done that day. He would listen for 15 minutes and then dismiss her. No longer living for the future, she clung to the past with its old resentments that caused pain and misunderstandings. She still cherished bitter feelings about her sisters' disapproval. As a child she had shrugged it off, but its continuance in adult years evoked angry response from her, and she became equally, if not more, critical of them. It was as if the unfathomable depths of resentment, envy, and jealousy that haunt the human heart flared up in sheer spite. Now in old age, Ethel's daughter, on whose care Eunice depended, became the target of what seemed to her malicious attacks on her mother, and her care for her aunt became reluctant. Eunice's friends, unaware of these strains, recoiled from her seeming lack of concern for her aunt's happiness. "She even refused to bring Miss Dyke to a birthday party I had planned for her," recalls one of them. So malice spawned further ill-feelings.

In the past similar reaction often marred Miss Dyke's relationships with her nurses and other colleagues. Yet through all the chance and change of living, the memory of her early mentor in the Department of Public Health shone like a beacon to the end. Dr. Hastings' daughter was moved to tears when she visited at 'Twin Elms' to have Miss Dyke ask, "Mrs. Williams, if I get all the nurses together, would you come and talk to us like your father used to do?"

After little more than three years in the nursing home, the last few months confined to bed, she died alone in an alien atmosphere. Miss Dyke was buried in the Dyke family plot in the Mount Pleasant Cementery in Toronto. A member of the Society of Friends presided over a grave-side service for her. A month or two after her death, the Society of Friends held a memorial service for her that brought relatives and friends, many of them for the first time, into a Quaker milieu. There were moving tributes to Miss Dyke, but it was not a solemn meeting. Several nurses told about amusing incidents that had occurred in the Nursing Division in her day, and there were tales of her delight in a practical joke. Those who remember the informality and friendliness of the occasion thought that Miss Dyke would have enjoyed it.

233

The Quondam Club, an organization of retired public health nurses, remember her also, and Dr. Florence Emory spoke for the group, many of whom, like her, had worked under Miss Dyke's leadership:

> At this meeting of the Quondam Club, 16 October 1969, members present wish to record their sense of individual and corporate loss in the recent death of Miss Eunice H. Dyke.

Dr. Emory referred to Miss Dyke's contribution, as first Director of the Division of Public Health Nursing of the Toronto Department of Public Health and to the development of the Division's work, enlarging on her leadership in maintaining high professional standards and mentioning achievements already noted in the citation read before the Canadian Public Health Association. Then she continued:

> As is often the case, Miss Dyke's success was made possible through acceptance of her recommendations by another: Medical Officer of Health, Dr. J.C.O. Hastings ... It was he who found "the sinews of war" to finance the remarkable growth of the Division of Public Health Nursing, speaking often of its members as 'les nurses'.
>
> It is fitting that this Club should thus pay tribute to a nurse who upheld the ideals of the organized profession in Canada, instilling in those for whose work she was responsible a lively interest in all matters concerned with local, provincial and national nursing education and services.
>
> Moreover, Miss Dyke had a second pioneer effort to her credit. Possessing a deep ingrained social sense, she established close working relationships with community social agencies as well as with existing health organizations so that when opportunity came in later professional life, she was the moving spirit in establishing Second Mile Clubs for senior citizens throughout the city. These have enriched the lives of untold numbers of elderly persons.
>
> It is not surprising, therefore, that some years ago Miss Dyke's outstanding contributions and signal services in the promotion of public health were recognized by the Canadian Public Health Association in conferring upon her honorary life membership in that body.[1]

Her life's journey had ended.

She had known insecurity and wrestled with defeat. Lack of artistry in human relationships had often marred her dealings with people. She had been an outsider in the cause of political rights for women to which so many of her contemporaries devoted their energies. Her ideas of men-women relations were distinctly Victorian. Yet her achievements stand unchallenged. She was the "woman of her time in the development of public health nursing, a true pioneer", recalled a public health nurse of a later period. She was germinating ideas for geriatric care well before the helping professions, let alone society as a whole, recognized the need for knowledge and skills having to do with ageing and the problems of the elderly. She discovered her métier and, endowed with creative capacity, pursued it with singlemindedness. Furthermore, she had become increasingly interested in politics, acquired a world view of the human condition and sought the ways of peace. Canons of judgment change with the passing of time and the exigencies of social change. Yet, although there are to this day as many opinions of Eunice Dyke as there are people who knew her, none disputes that she was "ahead of her time".

Notes

Prologue

1. P.H. Bryce, "History of Public Health in Canada". *The Canadian Therapeutic and Sanitary Engineer* I, 6. June 1910. pp. 287-291.
2. Geoffrey Bilson, *A Darkened House– Cholera in Nineteenth-Century Canada*, University of Toronto Press, 1980. Chapter 3, "Nothing to be heard but the 'Cholera' ': Upper Canada 1832, pp. 52-69.
3. Rev. C. Dade, M.A. "Notes on the Cholera Seasons of 1832 and 1834". (The results of personal observation.) *The Canadian Journal of Industry, Science and Art*: The Canadian Institute, Toronto. New Series, No. xxxvii, January 1862, p. 17.
4. Charles M. Godfrey, *The Cholera Epidemics in Upper Canada 1832-1866*. Seccombe House, Toronto and Montreal, 1968, p. 37.
5. *Upper Canada House of Assembly Journals– 1832-1833* . Appendix, p. 83. "Circular Addressed by the Government to the Chairmen of Quarter Sessions of Several Districts, on the breaking out of the Cholera", 20 June 1832.
6. *Upper Canada Statutes*, 1833. C. 47. (An Act to establish Boards of Health, and to guard against the introduction of malignant, contagious and infectious diseases in this Province.)
7. *Ibid.*, 1834. C. 23. An Act to extend the limits of the Town of York; to erect said Town into a City; and to Incorporate it under the name of the City of Toronto.
8. "The Act Concerning Nuisance and Good Government of the City" passed 30 March 1834. Signed by Wm. L. MacKenzie. *Journal of the Common Council of the City of Toronto*, 1834. April to August. City Clerk's Register of By-laws, 1834-1839. City of Toronto Archives. (C.T.A.)
9. *Ibid.*, An Act to establish a Board of Health, passed 9 June 1834.
10. Dade, p. 24.
11. Report of the Board of Health To the Mayor, Aldermen and Commonality of the City of Toronto, in Common Council Assembled. Quoted by William Canniff, *Medical Profession in Upper Canada*, Part II, pp. 80-82.
12. William Perkins Bull, *From Medicine Man to Medical Man*, The Perkins Bull Foundation, McLeod, 1914. Chapter V "From Plague and Pestilence". p. 90. ff.
13. *Statutes*, 1835. C. 15.
14. *Statutes*, 1839, C. 21.
15. *Statutes of Province of Canada*. 1849. C. 8.
16. Bull, p. 97.
17. *Ontario Statutes*, 1882. C. 38.
18. R.D. Defries, Ed. *The Development of Public Health in Canada*, University of Toronto Press, 1940, Preface p. viii.
19. *Statutes*, 1884, C. 38.
20. Bull, p. 244.
21. Robert Wilson, *A Retrospect*, A Short Review of the steps taken in Sanitation to transfer the Town of Muddy York into the Queen City of the West. Department of Public Health, City of Toronto, 1934. Canniff's contribution to sanitary reform and public health in Toronto is described at length, pp. 19-28 of the pamphlet.
22. *The Canadian Medical Association Journal*, New Series, xx, 1929. p. 449.
23. *The Globe*, Toronto. 2 May, p. 7 and 4 May, p. 12, 1900.
24. Adam H. Wright to his Worship the Mayor, Board of Control and Members of the City Council. Toronto, 7 October 1910. RG 1, Council Papers, 1910. (C.T.A.)

25. Christina Mitchell "Chronic Tuberculosis" in *The Canadian Nurse*, Vol. 3, No. 2, 1907.

26. Ernest Wills, "Sanitary Treatment and Early Diagnosis of Pulmonary Tuberculosis", *The Canadian Practitioner and Review*, xxix, 6, pp. 272, 274, 275.

27. The National Sanatorium Association, organized by Sir William Gage, had been granted a Dominion of Canada Charter in April 1896. Under its auspices, the Muskoka Cottage Hospital, the first sanatorium in Canada, was opened in July 1897. Brink, G.C. *Across the Years. Tuberculosis in Ontario*: Ontario Tuberculosis Association, 1965, p. 49.

28. The Sisters of St. Joseph belonged to an Order that had been founded in 1648 in France. Dissolved during the French Revolution, it was revived in 1778, and in 1836 a group of Sisters were sent to North America, first to the United States, and, in 1851, at the request of Bishop de Charbonnel, to Toronto. When the House of Providence was first opened in Power Street (near Queen and Parliament Streets), four or five nurses were assigned to the project. With slender means at their disposal, they went out begging to obtain support. In the countryside they asked for produce to provide food for those in their care. An institution with a long history of charitable work, now at 3276 St. Clair Avenue East, Toronto, and known as Providence Villa and Hospital, it is accredited for long-term care of the incurably ill. Information provided by the Director, Sister Liguori.

29. *The Globe*, Toronto, 10 and 11 December 1901. *The Evening News*, 10 December 1901.

30. Brink, p. 49.

31. Harvey Cushing, *The Life of William Osler*; Oxford. London, New York, Toronto. 1940, pp. 535-536. Referring to an address on 'The Healing of Tuberculosis' given by Osler at the Annual Meeting of the Maryland Medical and Chirugical Faculty on 30 April 1891, Cushing. p. 348, quotes Dr. W.H. Welch as having written: "Osler was perhaps the first to work out home treatment of tuberculosis".

32. Mary M. Roberts, *American Nursing– History and Interpretation*: MacMillan, New York, 1954.

33. Theodore B. Sachs, "The Tuberculosis Nurse", *The American Journal of Nursing*, viii, May 1908. pp. 597-598.

34. Population statistics based on assessment rolls, provided by C.T.A.

35. W.G. Cosbie, *The Toronto General Hospital, 1819-1956 – A Chronicle*: MacMillan. Toronto, 1975. p. 129.

36. Information provided by Mrs. Myrna Sclater, Director, the Division of Public Health Nursing, Toronto Department of Public Health, 1969 to 1977.

37. Cosbie, pp. 129-130.

38. City Council Minutes, Toronto, 8 July 1907.

39. "The Brown Book" Miss Dyke's handwritten records of the early days of the Division of Public Health Nursing. RG 11, F1, Box 5, City of Toronto Archives (C.T.A.) p. 4.

40. Brink, p. 56.

41. National Sanatorium Association. *Annual Report* 1908-1909, p. 22. "Report of the Visiting Nurse, C.L. Creighton, for the year ended 30 September 1909". She had visited 1,019 patients, sent 39 to the free hospitals (Weston and Muskoka) and had 52 homes disinfected. As well as looking after the sick, she had members of their families who had been exposed to the disease examined and had taken steps to prevent spread of the disease.

42. National Sanatorium Association. Annual Report, 1912-1913, p. 39. Miss Stewart did distinguished work in this post until her retirement which is reported in the *Annual Report, 1928-1929*, p. 43. Miss Violet Carroll who was appointed to the Public Health Nursing Division in 1917 recalled that Miss Stewart worked in close collaboration with the 'city nurses'.

43. Brink, pp. 41-42.

44. Katherine McCuaig, "From Social Reform to Social Service: The changing role of Volunteers; the Anti-Tuberculosis Campaign, 1900-1930". *Canadian Historical Review*, 1xi, 4 December 1980, pp. 480-501.

45. C.J.O. Hastings, "The Duty of the Profession and State Regarding the Mental and Physical Care of Improperly Cared-for Children". *The Canadian Practitioner and Review*, Toronto, vol. xxx, No. 7, July 1905, p. 368.
46. Dr. Hastings' daughter, Mrs. Audrey Williams, interviewed by the author. Also, Adam H. Wright to His Worship the Mayor, Board of Control, and Members of the City Council, Toronto.
47. John S. McCullough, "Obituary, Dr. Charles J.O. Hastings, Medical Officer of Health, Toronto, 1910-1929". *Canadian Public Health Journal*, vol. xxii, 1931, p. 159.
48. An anecdote recalled by a social worker who admired Dr. Hastings and remembers his reputation for vigorous action.
49. Dr. Hastings' opinion as expressed in a report of the Toronto Bureau of Municipal Research: Horace L. Brittain, "The Administration of the Toronto Department of Health", *The Public Health Journal*, Toronto, vi, No. 7, August 1917, p. 310.
50. Charles J. Hastings, "The Modern Conception of Public Health and Its National Importance", *The Canadian Medical Association Journal*, vii, No. 8, August 1917, p. 692.
51. Jesse Edgar Middleton, *The Municipality of Toronto – A History*. Dominion Publishing Company, Toronto and New York, 1923, p. 777.
52. "Report No. 8 of the Local Board of Health". *City of Toronto Council Minutes*. 1910. Appendix A. pp. 1365-1367. C.T.A.
53. C.J.O. Hastings, "Slum Conditions in Toronto", Medical Health Officer's Report, Department of Health, Toronto, 1911. No. 1-1-04. Folio No. 5, C.T.A.
54. Hastings. *The Canadian Medical Association Journal*, vol. vii, No. 8, August 1917, p. 690.
55. *The Toronto Daily Star*, 6 July to 20 August 1912.
56. Report of the Medical Officer of Health, November 1914. C.T.A.

Chapter One: Eunice Henrietta Dyke

1. C.-E.A. Winslow, "Nurses Show The Way". *Survey Graphic*, xxiii, 4 April 1934.
2. Miss Dyke's nieces, Miss Jean West and Mrs. Catherine Barrick, provided information about her family background. Rev. Dyke's career was reviewed in *The Canadian Baptist*, 28 May 1931. McMaster University Archives. Genealogical data was supplemented by Mr. Frank R. Stone of Toronto and Mr. Ross Ryrie of Oakville, Ontario.
3. Mary Millman, recently retired from the faculty of the University of Toronto School of Nursing, spent some years as a public health nurse under Miss Dyke's leadership in the Department of Public Health.
4. See Barbara J. Harris, *Beyond her Sphere– Women in the Professions in American History*, Greenwood. Westport, Connecticut, 1978, pp. 97-98.
5. Miss Hampton resigned in 1894, when she married Hunter Robb, Professor of Gynaecology, Western Reserve University, Cleveland, Ohio. Later she took an active part in organizing the International Council of Nurses. Miss Nutting resigned in 1907 on appointment to the staff of Columbia University. She was the first nurse to become a university professor.
6. Ethel Johns and Blanche Pfefferhorn, *The Johns Hopkins School of Nursing, 1889-1949*. The Johns Hopkins Press, Baltimore, 1954.
7. An association confirmed by Dr. Hastings' daughter, Mrs. Audrey Williams.

Chapter Two: A Mammoth Undertaking

1. Florence Emory began her career in public health nursing when she joined Miss Dyke's staff in 1915. In 1923, she was awarded a fellowship by the American Child Health Association and granted leave for study at Simmons College, Boston, with lectures also at M.I.T. On returning to Toronto she was appointed to the staff of the newly organized Department of Nursing of the University of Toronto. She is the author of *Public Health Nursing in Canada*, a comprehensive study of the subject, first published in 1949 and for decades used as a textbook in schools of nursing. Miss Emory is a past president of the Registered Nurses' Association of Ontario.
2. G.C. Brink, *Across the Years, Tuberculosis in Ontario*. Ontario Tuberculosis Association, 1965. pp. 42, 43.
3. Charles J. Hastings, M.D., "Nursing Organization as Developed in Toronto", *The Nation's Health*, Chicago, 15 February 1923, p. 62.
4. *The Canadian Nurse*, XIII, 1917, p. 121.
5. *Statistical Review*, Department of Public Health, City of Toronto, 1934, T.C.A.
6. Enid Forsythe, "Child Welfare Clinics", *The Canadian Nurse*, XIII, 1917, p. 621.
7. Michael J. Piva, *The Condition of the Working Class in Toronto, 1900-1921*, University of Ottawa Press, 1979, pp. 121-125.
8. Forsythe, P. 622.
9. Horace L. Brittain, Director, Toronto Bureau of Municipal Research, "Administration of the Toronto Department of Health", *The Public Health Journal*, Toronto, Canada. vi, No. 8, July 1915. pp. 365-377, deals with the Division of Public Health Nurses.
10. *The Labour Gazette*, Department of Labour, Ottawa, August 1914, p. 187.
11. For a sketch of Brown's career, see Dorothy Sangster, "Alan Brown of Sick Kids", *Maclean's Magazine*, August 1952.
12. Alan Brown, M.D., "Infant and Child Welfare Work". *The Canadian Public Health Journal*, April 1918, vol. ix, No. 4.
13. Paul Adolphus Bator, "The Struggle to Raise the Lower Classes: Public Health Reform and Problem of Poverty in Toronto, 1910-1921". *Journal of Canadian Studies*, XIV, no. 1, Spring 1979, p. 400. Bator points out that the N.W.A. originated in response to the efforts of the Department of Public Health to cope with financial causes of ill health.
14. F.N. Stapleford, *After Twenty Years, A Short History of the Neighborhood Workers' Association, 1918-1938*. Neighborhood Workers' Association (N.W.A.) Toronto, 1938, p. 7.
15. N.W.A., "Statement of Policy. Beginnings of the Association", n.d. (probably written about 1934). Papers of Ethel Dodds Parker entrusted to A. Harriet Parsons.
16. A. Harriet Parsons, "The Role of J.J. Kelso in the Canadian Settlement Movement". Unpublished paper, 1978. Burnett applied for the post of Superintendent of the University Settlement in Toronto in a letter to President Falconer, written in New York, March 10, 1913. Falconer Papers, Box 26, University of Toronto Archives.
17. Report of the Medical Officer of Health to the Board of Health, August 1915, adopted by the Board, September 15, 1915 and Parker, "N.W.A. Statement of Policy".
18. "Social Service Commission. A report dealing with the origin, dates, growth and work since November 1912". Signed: Edwin Dickie, Secretary, Social Service Commission, Toronto, 1 March 1921. 34. pp. C.T.A.

19. Papers of Ethel Dodds Parker.

20. "An Act to Regulate Maternity Boarding Houses and for the Protection of Infant Children", 1887. *Revised Statutes of Ontario, 1897*, 2. C258, 60 V., C. 52, 514. "The Maternity Boarding House Act". 1914 Revised Statutes of Ontario, 1914, 2.C230, Geo. V., C. 60. S1., sections 5-12 (inclu.) defined the responsibility of the local medical officer of health more precisely than the original legislation. He was to be satisfied that the house was suitable to be registered and that the applicant for registration was of good character and "able to maintain, help and properly lodge women or girls or infants". (Allan M. Dymond, *The Laws of Ontario Relating to Women and Children*, Toronto. Clarkson W. James, 1923, p. 79.

21. Mary Stirritt, "Child Placing". *The Canadian Nurse*, 13: 8, 1917 pp. 478, 479.

Chapter Three: Fresh Challenges

1. "History of the Division of Public Health Nursing". An outline of the work of the Division of Public Health Nursing, Department of Public Health, Toronto, 1939. Anonymous. C.T.A., RG11, F1.

2. Dominion Bureau of Statistics, *Census Canada, 1911*. Out of a population of 374,667 in Toronto, the census reported 17,713 Jews and 4,197 Italians. Other European immigrants were so grouped as to be indistinguishable by nationality. The number of Chinese was 1,036. Robert Harney and Harold Troper, *Immigrants: A Portrait of Urban Experience*, 1890-1930. Van Nostrand, Reinhold, Toronto, 1975.

3. *The Labour Gazette*, 19 March 1915, p. 1060.

4. "History of the Division of Public Health Nursing, 1939".

5. L. Petroff. "Macedonians from Village to City". An interview with Mr. and Mrs. F. Tornev, February 1976. *Canadian Ethnic Studies*, xi, 1, 1977, p. 37.

6. Harney and Troper, p. 138.

7. Neil Sutherland, "To create a strong and healthy race in school children in the public health movement, 1880-1914". *History of Education Quarterly*, xii, 3, 1972, p. 318.

8. Keefer, p. 6.

9. Lina Roger, *The School Nurse*, Putman, New York, 1917. pp. 38-46.

10. Interview with Mary Millman, 4 January 1979.

11. Charles J.C.O. Hastings, "Medical Inspection of Public Schools", *Canadian Journal of Medicine and Surgery*, 21, 1907, p. 73.

12. Florence Helen Emory. *Public Health Nursing in Canada*, Macmillan, Toronto, 1945. p. 167.

13. Cyril Greenland, "Services for the Mentally Retarded in Ontario, 1870-1930", *Ontario History*, Vol. LIV(1962), No. 4.

14. Report of Special Committee in Medical Inspection Department, *Annual Report of the Toronto Board of Education*, 1912. Appendix, p. 939.

15. *A Brief History of the Ontario Welfare Council, 1908-1959*. Ontario Welfare Council, Toronto, Canada. p. 5.

16. W.G. Cosbie, *The Toronto General Hospital– 1819-1965: A Chronicle*, MacMillan, Toronto. 1975. p. 160.

17. Keefer, p. 6.

18. *Report of the Department of Labour for the fiscal year ending, 31 March 1912*. King's Printer, Ottawa, pp. 7-8.

19. *Board of Control Minutes, July-Dec., 1920*. Minute No. 1344.

20. Board of Health Report No. 6., 7 March 1921.

21. Stapleford, *After Twenty Years*, p. 19.

22. Robert E. Mills, "Hospital Social Service as a Community Problem– The Toronto Plan", *Hospital Social Service*, Vol. 3, Jan. 1921, pp. 55-62.

23. Bator, For discussion of the burden of 'poor relief' carried by the Department of Health and its consequences, pp. 43 ff.

24. *City Council Minutes*, Toronto, 1921. Vol. 2., Appendix A, p. 989.

25. Hastings, *The Nation's Health*, 1923, p. 63.

26. *Ibid.*, p. 65.

27. Report of the Medical Office of Health, February 1919. Also recorded in a letter written by Hastings to Sir Robert Falconer, President of the University of Toronto, 3 June 1920. Falconer Papers U. of T. Archives.

Chapter Four: An International Figure

1. *Encyclopaedia Britannica*, Vol. 19, 1966. pp. 26-27. Any edition of the encyclopaedia gives an account of the origins of the Red Cross, including the International Committee and the League of Red Cross Societies.
2. Herbert Henry Asquith, as leader of the Liberal Party had been Prime Minister of Britain from 1908 to 1916.
3. A brochure of the Cowdray Club, undated, in the archives of a library in Baker Street in London described the Club and lists the distinguished women who, over the years, served as vice-presidents. In mid-1960's, to counteract a decline in membership, men were admitted, and in the early 1970's, it merged with the Naval and Military Club in Piccadilly.
4. "List of Training Centres Aided by the Rockefeller Foundation", G AA/MB, 4 April 1924, among Miss Dyke's papers.
5. Recommendation attached to letter to Olmsted, 9 April 1924.
6. "England". Miss Dyke's report of her experiences, supplemented by comments in her letter to Dr. Hastings, is the source of the information.
7. "Minutes of the Meeting of the Executive Committee of the Canadian Red Cross Society, 1 February 1924". The motion was made by Mrs. Plumptre and seconded by Col. Nasmith.
8. E. Kathleen Russell, Director, Department of Public Health Nursing, University of Toronto, to Miss Dyke, c/o League of Red Cross Societies, Paris. 8 February 1924. Nora Moore was acting head of the Division of Public Nursing in the Toronto Department of Public Health, during Miss Dyke's absence.
9. An observation of one of Miss Russell's colleagues who knew both women.

Chapter Five: After Paris

1. An outline history of the division of public health nursing, 1944. RG 11, F 1, Box 4, C.T.A. In January 1929, Hastings had reported the existence of 1,667 clinics with an attendance of more than 47,000.
2. Samples of these pamphlets have been deposited in the City Archives, C.T.A. RG11, F1, Box 7.
3. Marjorie Bell, *Visiting Homemakers' Association*, 1921-1949. Unpublished paper in archives of the Association. Bell was the director from 1932 to 1945; Canadian Red Cross Society (C.R.S.), *Minutes of the Central Council*, 22, 23 November 1965. (A review and evaluation of the Society's homemaker service, C.R.S., Ontario Division, 1949), and *Papers of the Canadian Welfare Council*, "Information for a Synopsis of Provincial Reports in Progress in Public Health Nursing in Canada, 1924-26", Correspondence of the Canadian Nurses' Association with the Canadian Council on Child Welfare, 1926. MG 28, 1, 10, Vol. 28. File No. 140, P.A.C; "The duties of Visiting Homemakers", *The Canadian Nurse*, XXXIII, 3, March 1937, pp. 125-126, an article based on a letter from Eunice Dyke in which she described the Toronto Homemakers' Association as a useful forum for evaluation of community services of varied purpose and type.
4. Report of the Medical Officer of Health, No. 1, 1927. *City Council Minutes*, 1927. Appendix A, pp. 92-98; Re 'polio', see Samuel Benison, "Poliomyelitis and the Rockefeller Institute: Social Effects and Institutional Response", *Journal of History of Medicine and Allied Sciences*, XXIX, January 1974, pp. 74-92.

5. Keefer, p. 8.
6. Department of Public Health, Toronto. *Report of the Medical Officer of Health.* April and September, 1920. See also Hastings, *The Nation's Health*, p. 64.
7. *Survey of Family Social Work Field of Toronto, Canada.* Under the auspices of the Federation for Community Service, by Frances H. McLean Field Director, and Ruth Hill, Associate, American Organization for Organizing Family Social Work and Margaret V. Nairn (Volunteer), 1927. Archives of the Family Service Association of Metropolitan Toronto.
8. Outline history of public health nursing division.
9. The Charter of the Canadian Association of Social Workers was issued in 1926; local chapters were formed in Montreal, in 1927, and in Toronto, in 1928. In both cities there had been earlier informal groups.
10. Eunice Dyke, "The Canadian Nurses' Association and the National Council of Women of Canada", *The Canadian Nurse*, XXIII, 6, June 1927, pp. 301-303.
11. Keefer, p. 6, and Papers of the *Canadian Welfare Council*, File No. 178, P.A.C.
12. *The Toronto Daily Star*, Saturday, 9 May 1931, announced the meeting and listed the speakers. Among them were Dr. Helen MacMurchy, doctors Jackson and Robb for the Department of Public Health and Mayor Stewart.
13. Report of the Advisory Committee to Local Board of Health on Maternal Welfare, adopted by the Corporation of the City of Toronto, June 1933. Department of Public Health, Toronto. Report No. 7, C.T.A. The September 30 meeting was described in *The Toronto Daily Star*, 1 October 1931, p. 14.
14. *City Council Minutes, Toronto*, 1931. Vol. I. Appendix A, p. 1680.

Chapter Six: The Consuming Concern

1. Information gleaned from conversation with Eileen Cryderman, a younger member of Miss Dyke's staff who later became Director of the Division of Public Health Nursing. Miss Dyke's philosophy of team play is explained in an article entitled "Team Play for Health", *The Canadian Nurse*, 15, Dec. 1919. pp. 2175-2180, and Dr. Hastings comment occurs in his article in *The Nation's Health*, Chicago, 1923, p. 64.
2. "Division of Public Health Nursing, Department of Public Health. Toronto. General statement of purpose and organization", dated March 1934, RG11 F1 Box 4, C.T.A. In a letter to Hastings, 8 February 1917, Miss Dyke informed him of the nurses' request that she refer to him "a question from the question box", an action that she considered 'exceptional' on the part of any group of nurses.
3. Outline of history of the Division of Public Health Nursing.
4. Report of the Medical Officer of Health, June 1917. Section contributed by the Division of Social Service. C.T.A.
5. *Falconer Papers*, University of Toronto Archives, A66. 003 35. Box 32. The prospectus was published in *The Canadian Nurse*, Toronto, September 1914, No. 9, pp. 525-528:
6. Notes on the history of the Division of Public Health Nursing, written by Dyke. RG11, F1, Box 4. C.T.A.
7. A bulletin from the Reference Library of Simmons College, obtained in 1974, through the courtesy of Christine Viano, Assistant Reference Librarian of the College, was the source of information about the Course.
8. Petition addressed to President Falconer and a resolution from the alumni of the Department, both dated 2 June 1919, Falconer Papers, Box 53, University of Toronto Archives.
9. Mary Stirritt, "Child Placing", *The Canadian Nurse*, 13, 8, 1917, p. 477-481; and Enid Forsythe, "Child Welfare Clinics", *The Canadian Nurse*, 13, 10, 1917, pp. 621-625.
10. Zada Keefer, Ed. "The History of Public Health Nursing in Toronto", 1945. p. 6. Unpublished paper, C.T.A., RG. 11, F1, Box 4.

11. R.M. MacIver, Director, University of Toronto, Department of Social Service to Sir Robert Falconer, 4 December 1919. University of Toronto Archives, *Falconer Papers*, Box 59. A further memo dated 10 Dec. recommended an honorarium of $400 for Kathleen Russell as a lecturer in the Department.
12. Source: "The Role of One Voluntary Organization in Canada's Health Service". A Brief presented to the Royal Commission on Health Services on behalf of the Central Council of the Canadian Red Cross Society, May 1962. Chapter VIII, Nursing Education, 96ff. National Office, The Canadian Red Cross Society, Toronto.
13. "Public Health Nursing", *Falconer Papers*.
14. "The Division of Public Health Nursing".
15. *Falconer Papers*, In addition to those from the Department of Public Health, there were 14 from the Victorian Order, three from the Government Department of Soldiers' Civil Reestablishment and six listed as Miscellaneous.
16. Edith Kathleen Russell, "The Training of a Public Health Nurse". *The World's Health*, October 1928. Later published in *The Canadian Nurse*. See also by the same author, "Public Health Field Work for the Undergraduate Nurse", *The Canadian Nurse*, August 1920, and "Public Health Nursing Education and the Undergraduate Nurse", *The Canadian Nurse*, November 1926.
17. "The Division of Public Health Nursing".
18. Notes on the history of the Division prepared by Miss Dyke.

Chapter Seven: Arousing Public Awareness

1. "History of the Graduate Nurses Association of Ontario", *The Canadian Nurse*, IX, 5, May 1913, pp. 296-306.
2. "Milestone to the Present", *The Leaf and the Lamp*, Canadian Nurses Association, Ottawa, 1968, p. 83. (In 1917 the Canadian Society of Superintendents of Training Schools for Nurses changed its name to the Canadian Association of Nursing Education).
3. "Report of Special Committee on Nurse Education", *The Canadian Nurse*, X, 10, October 1914, pp. 570-580.
4. Eunice H. Dyke, "The Organization of Public Health Nursing". Read before Canadian Conference on Charities and Correction, Ottawa, 1917. *The Canadian Nurse*, Vol. XIV, May 1918, p. 1017. It is worth noting that it was in 1973 that the Ontario Ministry of Education accepted responsibility for nursing education within the curriculum of the community colleges of the Province.
5. Falconer Papers, Box 53.
6. *The Canadian Nurse*, IX, 1913, p. 612.
7. *Ibid.*, X, 10, 1914.
8. *The Public Health Journal*, Toronto, Vol. VI, January, February, March 1915.
9. Hastings to Falconer, 3 June 1920. Papers of President Falconer, University of Toronto Archives.
10. Eunice H. Dyke, "The Organization of Public Health Nursing", *The Canadian Nurse*, Vol. XIV, May 1918, pp. 1017-1019.
11. *Ibid.*, "Team Play for Health", *The Canadian Nurse*, XV, pp. 2175-2180, December 1919.
12. *The Canadian Nurse*, XIII, 8, August 1917, pp. 420-422.
13. Minutes of the Seventh General Meeting of the CNATN, 6-8 June 1918, West Hall, University of Toronto, Archives of the Canadian Nurses Association (CNA), Ottawa.
14. Minutes of the Eighth General Meeting of the CNATN, Vancouver July 1919, CNA Archives.
15. Minutes of Ninth General Meeting of CNATN, afternoon session, 5 July 1920.
16. Proceedings of the Public Health Meetings of the CNATN (after 1924 the CNA) in particular 1921, 1925, 1926 and 1932. Archives of CNA.

17. Minutes of the Meeting of the Board of Directors of the CNATN, June 1919, Archives of CNA.
18. The Canadian Red Cross Society, "The Role of One Voluntary Organization in Canada's Health Service". A Brief presented on behalf of the Central Council of the Canada's Red Cross Society to the Royal Commission on Health Services, May 1962. Chapter VIII. "Nursing Education", p. 96.
19. Eunice H. Dyke, "What has been Accomplished by the Committee on National Nursing Service". *The Canadian Nurse*, XV, 11, 1919, pp. 2111, 2112.
20. Minutes of the Tenth General Meeting of the CNATN, Quebec, 1-4 June, 1921, p. 61, Archives of CNA.
21. Information from Canadian Nurses' Association archival records made available by the Librarian, Margaret Parkin.
22. Eunice H. Dyke, "Public Health Nursing", *The Canadian Nurse*, XXIII, 9, September 1927, pp. 479-483. Details of the four-year course offered by the University Department of Nursing were provided in an unpublished paper by Dr. Helen Carpenter, a tribute to Dr. Kathleen Russell.
23. George M. Weir, *Survey of Nursing Education in Canada*, Toronto. University of Toronto Press, 1932.
24. Eunice Dyke, "Survey of Nursing Education in Canada– The Implications for Public Health Nurses". *The Canadian Nurse*, XXVIII, 10, October 1932.

Chapter Eight: Collapse of a Career

1. The episode is described in a statement from the Registered Nurses Association addressed to Mayor William Stewart and published in *The Toronto Daily Star*, 7 October 1932; in a communication from Godfrey and Corcoran, Barristers, dated 28 October, also addressed to the Mayor. Minutes of the City Council, 31 October 1932. 779, and in the Judgment of Judge O'Connell in the case of Mary E. Bullick vs The Corporation of the City of Toronto, delivered in December 1932. City of Toronto Archives (C.T.A.)
2. Minutes of the Board of Control, 20 July 1932, 262.
3. *The Toronto Daily Star*, also *The Globe*, Toronto, 7 October 1932.
4. *The Globe*, 10 October 1932.
5. Judge O'Connell, p. 3.
6. *The Toronto Daily Star*, 8 October 1932, p. 3.
7. Jackson to Mayor Stewart and Members of the Board of Control, 1193, L b15. C.T.A.
8. *The Toronto Daily Star*, 7 October 1932.
9. Godfrey and Corcoran, Barristers.
10. Minutes of the City Council, 28 November 1932, 884.
11. M.E. Maitland, Prince's Lake, Ontario, to Mayor Stewart, 10 November 1932.
12. County Court of the County of York, Mary E. Bullick vs. The Corporation of the City of Toronto, *Judgment*, pp. 17, 24, 25 and 26. C.T.A. Minutes of the City Council, 13 December 1932. 954, 956, 957, 958 and 959.
13. Jackson to Mayor Stewart and members of the Board of Control, 1 February 1933. Board of Control Minutes, 1 February 1933, 369. Although Jackson's letter was filed, the Kenny letter has not been kept. "Charlie Millar's Million Dollar Joke", *MacLean's*, v. 16, 15 June 1952, pp. 18-19, 26.
14. The O'Connell Judgment, 3 January 1933. pp. 10-11.
15. *The Toronto Daily Star*, 2 February 1933, citing remarks of Barbara Blackstock, and 3 February quoting a letter from Mrs. Hynes to all members of the City Council.
16. *The Globe*. 2 February 1933. Editorial, "A Dangerous Principle".
17. Anna P. Meldrum to the Mayor and City Council, Toronto. 3 February 1933.
18. M.A. Gibson to Observer, Care Daily Star, 1 February 1933. Minutes of the City Council, 6 February 1933. 132.

19. *The Toronto Daily Star*, 7 February 1933. p. 6.
20. *The Globe*, Toronto, 8 February 1933. Editorial, "The Council was Right".

Chapter Nine: A Rockefeller Fellowship

1. *The Toronto Daily Star*. 6 May 1933. *The Globe* and *The Telegram* of the same date. Also, Jean I. Gunn, "Honour where honour is due". *The Canadian Nurse*, xxix, 10 October 1933.
2. Tom Thomson, the first Canadian painter to portray the north country, who had drowned in 1917, had become a legend, and the Group of Seven, formed in 1919, had continued to open the eyes of Canadians to the rugged grandeur of our northern landscapes.
3. A.J. Warren, M.D. of the Rockefeller Foundation to Dyke, 23 August 1933.
4. Dyke to Frederick W. Russell, Director, International Health Division, Rockefeller Foundation, 12 September 1933.
5. This project is mentioned repeatedly in personal letters as well as in correspondence with Mary Beard and other individuals, including Dr. C.-E.A. Winslow of the School of Medicine, Yale University, New Haven, Conn.
6. Edward Robb Ellis, *A Nation in Torment, The Great American Depression, 1929-1939*. Coward-McCann, New York, 1970. C. 17, 'March 1933', pp. 255-287, also "Migrants and Civilian Conservation Corps", C. 18; "Droughts and Dust Storms, Ohio and Vigilantes", C. 26, and "Federal Emergency Relief Act creating FERA", C. 27.
7. *The Survey*, Survey Associates, New York, v. LXX, 5, 1934, p. 164.
8. *Ibid.* Grace Abbott, Chief, U.S. Children's Bureau, "Child Health Recovery". v. LXIX, 10, 1933.
9. Arthur Mann, *La Guardia: A Fighter Against His Times 1882-1933*. Lippincott, Philadelphia, 1965, and by the same author, *La Guardia Comes to Power, 1933*. Lippincott, 1965.
10 La Guardia's achievements were listed among subjects dealt with in a talk about her "sabbatical leave" that Miss Dyke gave before the Manitoba Association of Registered Nurses, in Winnipeg in May 1934.
11. *The New York Times*, 1 September 1957, p. 31. An account of Winslow's life and work written at the time of his death. For his concept of public health, see Reginald M. Atwater, "C.-E.A. Winslow, An Appreciation of a Great Statesman", *American Journal of Public Health*, 47, 9, 1957, pp. 1065-1070.
12. Held 14-15 March, at the New York Academy of Medicine. The Milbank Memorial Fund, which sponsored scientific research in public health and demography, had been established by Elizabeth Milbank Anderson, who inherited a large fortune from her father, Jeremiah Milbank, organizer and builder of the Chicago, Milwaukee and St. Paul Railroad.
13. *The Survey*. 1xx, 4, 126-127. See also Edgar Sydenstricker, "Sickness and the New Poor", *Survey Graphic*, New York, xxiii, 4, 160-162.
14. Dyke to Beard, 16 March 1934. In this letter Dyke quoted long passages from Whitton's letter, a complete copy of which is among Canadian Welfare Council papers in the Public Archives of Canada (P.C.A.) M 9 28, 4. (File 178).

Chapter Ten: Return to Canada

1. Mrs. A.W. Bailey. "The Year We Moved", *Pages from the Past, Essays in Saskatchewan History*, D.H. Bocking, Saskatoon, 1979. pp. 225-238.
2. T.C. Douglas, at the time minister of the Baptist Church in Weyburn, Sask., was a CCF candidate in the 1934 Saskatchewan election.
3. "Trachoma Report", Province of Saskatchewan, *Annual Report of the Department of Public Health*, 1934, p. 23. (Saskatchewan Archives Board).

4. It had been assumed that Dr. Fleming, as Deputy M.O.H., would be appointed to succeed Dr. Hastings, but his acceptance of the post in Montreal shortly before Dr. Hastings' retirement led to Dr. Jackson's appointment. Information provided by Florence Emory.

5. Whitton to Falk, 30 June 1934. Public Archives of Canada, Canadian Welfare Council Papers, MG 28 I 10. Canadian Council in Child and Family Welfare, Vol. 4, File No. 17. Child Hygiene Section. Correspondence. Miss Dyke, 1934.

Chapter Eleven: Six Months Trial

1. *Papers of the Canadian Welfare Council,* (CWC) MG 28, I. 10. Vol. 4, File 17. "Child Hygiene Secretaryship". Part 2, 1934. P.A.C.
2. *Ibid.* "Unfinished Business", July 1934.
3. *Ibid.* Vol. 39, File 168, 1934. "Minutes of the Treasury Board affecting transfer of services from the Division of Child Welfare of the Department of Health to the Council on Child and Family Welfare". After the transfer of services had been mutually agreed upon, the Constitution was re-cast, and the Council was incorporated under Letters Patent issued by the Secretary of State in May 1934.
4. *Ibid.* Vol. 41, File 168, "Child Health Section", Vol. 3, Part 2, 1934. "Minutes of the Meeting of the Executive of the Division on Child and Maternal Hygiene, 1 July 1934".
5. *Ibid.* Vol. 4, File 17, "Health Teaching Materials", 1934.
6. *The Canadian Nurse,* Vol. 30, 1934, "Dame Janet Campbell".
7. *CWC Papers,* Vol. 5, File 140, 1934, "Dame Janet Campbell".
8. *Ibid.,* Vol. 12, File 56. "Department of Immigration and Colonization", 1934.
9. *Ibid.,* Vol. 4, File 19, 1934. "Child Welfare Section", Vol. 3, 1934.
10. CWC Papers, Vol. 4, File 19, 1934.

Chapter Twelve: Further Ventures

1. *The Toronto Daily Star,* 16 January 1935. There are many accounts of social conditions in Toronto and environs, e.g. Patricia V. Schultz, *The East York Workers' Association, A Response to the Great Depression.* New Hogtown Press. Toronto, 1975; Bruce West, *Toronto,* Chap. 21, "The Depression Years", which confirm the author's recollections of the decade.
2. The Old Age Security Act, which came into effect 1 January 1952, created a universal old age pension of $40 per month with no means test, 20 years' residence being the only condition. As of 1 July 1957 the amount was increased to $46 a month, was raised again in November to $55 in 1962, to $65 and in October 1963 to $75.
3. *The Toronto Daily Star,* 23 January 1935.
4. *Report of the Lieutenant Governor's Commission on Housing Conditions in Toronto 1934* (signed by Herbert Bruce). Metro Toronto Municipal Library.
5. Roger E. Riendeau, "A Clash of Interests: Dependency and the Municipal Problem in the Great Depression", *Journal of Canadian Studies,* vol. 14, no. 1, Spring 1979, p. 50 ff.
6. Winifred Hutchison. *Report on Labour Conditions in Industries* in Toronto. Submitted to the Royal Commission on Price Spreads, and Mass Buying in January 1935. Public Archives of Canada, RG 33 b18. Vol. 93.
7. *The Toronto Daily Star,* 26 January 1935.
8. Patricia V. Schultz. *The East York Workers' Association. A Response to the Great Depression.* New Hogtown Press, Toronto. 1975. p. 51.
9. Ben. Holmes to the author, 8 June 1980.
10. Jean M. Good, "Fun at Sixty", *Canadian Welfare,* December 1947. Vol. xxiii.

11. Jean M. Good, "The Story of the Early Days of the Movement Which Led to the Second Mile Club of Toronto". Unpublished paper, n. d., provided by Mrs. Good.

12. Eunice Dyke to Jean Good, August 27, 1959.

13. An incident recalled by Mrs. Doreen Nolan, formerly Mrs. Corps.

14. City Council Minutes, Toronto, 1947. Board of Control Report II, 32, Appendix A. pp. 2057-2059. C.T.A.

15. Minutes of the Second Mile Club, 5 June 1947. Courtesy of the Headquarters Office, 110 Edward Street, Toronto.

16. *Ibid.* 16 June 1947.

Chapter Thirteen: A New Way of Life

1. Jean Good described this experience.

2. Minutes of Second Mile Club, 20 January 1948 – 5 March 1958.

3. Doreen Corps, after the death of her first husband married Carl Nolan, and now lives in Tucson, Arizona. She visited Toronto briefly in September 1980 and while in the city related the couple's association with Eunice Dyke. 9 September 1980.

4. Suzann Buckley, "Ladies or Midwives? Efforts to Reduce Infant and Maternal Mortality", Linda Kealey, *A Not Unreasonable Claim*, The Women's Press, 1979, pp. 142-149.

5. In 1936, *The Mail and Empire* merged with *The Globe* to become *The Globe and Mail*.

6. Dorothy Henderson, *Will Mankind Listen – A Tribute to Dr. Brock Chisholm*. Vancouver, 1970.

7. Based on information provided through Jean West and various present-day residents of Scarborough, obtained through the courtesy of George Barker, Chairman, Metropolitan Housing Company.

8. Charles M. Johnston, *McMaster University*. Vol. I, The Toronto Years. University of Toronto Press, Toronto. 1976, p. 172.

9. Conversation with Violet Carroll.

10. Information provided by Jean Good.

Chapter Fourteen: Her Last Days

1. Excerpted from Dr. Emory's manuscript which was obtained from the staff of Friends House, Lowther Avenue, Toronto.

The Dyke Family

| Rev. Samuel Allerthorn Dyke
2 Jun. 1845 – 6 Jun. 1931

m Jennie Ryrie
25 Jan. 1850 – 16 Jan. 1901 | Jennie Ethel Dyke
13 Dec. 1872 – 8 Aug. 1930

m Joseph MacDonald West
4 Dec. 1872 – 29 Mar. 1937

James Ethelbert Dyke
7 Mar. 1873 – 26 Apr. 1943

Margaret Winnifred Dyke
1 Sept. 1876 – 2 Sept. 1950

m John Fox
1 Sept. 1876 – 21 Jun. 1932

Samuel Allerthorn Dyke
25 Feb. 1880 – 20 Sept. 1943

m Catherine Lydia Stafford Jones
6 April 1883 – 27 Jul. 1953

Eunice Henrietta Dyke
8 Feb. 1883 – 1 Sept. 1969

Frederick Gordon Dyke
27 Dec. 1884 – 21 June 1931 | Thomas MacDonald West
27 Aug. 1899 – 5 Mar. 1972

Jean Ryrie West
22 Mar. 1902 – 28 Aug. 1982

John Holloway Fox
24 May 1903

Elizabeth Howard Fox
26 Nov. 1904 – 20 Aug. 1953

Catherine Marsden Fox
31 Oct. 1906 –

m C.G. Barrick
20 Nov. 1904 –

Joanne Allerthorn Fox
21 Oct. 1910 – 28 Dec. 1963 |

Partial Family Tree

248

The Ryrie Family

James Ryrie
1 Jan. 1817 – 9 Dec. 1888

m Margaret Piggott
1827 – 8 Feb. 1877

Daniel Ryrie
10 Feb. 1848 – 1 Jul. 1867

Jennie Ryrie
25 Jan. 1850 – 16 Jun. 1901

m Samuel Allerthorn Dyke
(see Dyke family)

Elizabeth (Bessie) Ryrie
17 Feb. 1852 – 6 Jun. 1896

m Nicholas Stambury Tarr
15 Dec. 1848 – 20 Jan. 1920

James Ryrie
21 April 1854 – 7 Jun. 1933

m Catherine McLean
12 Jun. 1855 – 27 Mar. 1927

Meta Ryrie
28 Apr. 1881 – 6 Feb. 1957

m John Edgar Stone
21 Mar. 1878 – 11 Mar. 1965

Son: Frank Reid Stone
31 Mar. 1909 –

Grace McLean Ryrie
6 Sept. 1898

m George Brock Chisholm
18 May 1896 – 2 Feb. 1971

William Piggott Ryrie
13 Oct. 1857 – Nov. 1919

Matilda (Aunt Tillie) Ryrie
2 Dec. 1859 – 6 Sept. 1910

m Robert Oliver Smith
1859 – 3 Oct. 1931

Harry Ryrie
9 May 1862 – 6 Sept. 1917

m Christine (Aunt Tina) Whittet
3 Jan. 1864 – 19 Mar. 1952

their youngest daughter
Margaret Ryrie
7 May 1899

m Gerald Alfred Birks
30 Oct. 1894

Ross Ryrie
10 Mar. 1901

Partial Family Tree

Illustration and Photograph Credits

Index

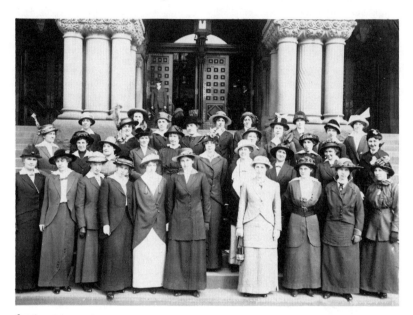

front cover

City of Toronto Department of Public Health Nurses 30 September 1914. Names of those known, starting on the left side.

First Row: 1-unknown, 2-unknown, 3-unknown, 4-Jessie Wood, 5-Daisey Halley, 6-Eunice Dyke, 7-unknown, 8-May Foy, 9-Ella Sutherland, 10-Miss Wells.

Second Row: 11-Miss McNeil, 12-unknown, 13-Betty Dingwall, 14-unknown, 15-unknown, 16-Enid Forsythe, 17-Agnes Milroy, 18-unknown, 19-unknown, 20-Miss McPherson.

Third Row: 21-unknown, 22-unknown, 23-unknown, 24-Edith Nisbet, 25-Dora Robinson, 26-Mabel Jewison, 27-Marjory Gardner, 28-Miss Lowther, 29-Thyra Jordon, 30-Miss Robb, 31-Edna Fraser, 32-Edna Blainey, 33-Gertrude O'Hara.